Soiled Linens

& Loved Ones

The Physical Act of Caregiving for the Non-Professional

By:

K. Rose Copeland

Caution: May Contain Profanity

Copyright © 2024 by **K. Rose Copeland**

All rights reserved. This book or any portion thereof may not be reproduced or used in any manner whatsoever without the express written permission of the publisher except for the use of brief quotations in a book review.

Printed in the United States of America

First Printing, 2024

ISBN: 9798874447588

Edited By R.S. Goings

rsg@aresge.com

Published By K. Rose Copeland

krosecopeland@gmail.com

Soiled Linens & Loved Ones

The Physical Act of Caregiving for the NON-Professional

By:

K. Rose Copeland

Caution: May Contain Profanity

Whether you are giving care, or receiving it, we will ALL

inevitably be in this position.

You will need this material on the physical and emotional
"GRUNT of CARING"

and "EVERYTHING" that comes with it.

CAUTION: MAY CONTAIN PROFANITY!

The choice of words used in this book may be frowned upon by many.

However, I grew up in a home that said, "Curse words are a form of expression and should ONLY be used for FEELING behind the message." NEVER curse at others!

Plus, I was told a genius swears.

Dedication

This is dedicated to everyone who tries to help someone.

You are Love.

Table of Contents

Introduction	8
Chapter 1: Getting To Know What You And Your Loved One Wants and Needs	21
Chapter 2: Universal Precautions - They're Coming Home!	43
Chapter 3: LOCC, Meals, Meds and Wound Care	65
Chapter 4: Medical Equipment & Devices	86
Chapter 5: Repositioning	105
Chapter 6: Transfer	122
Chapter 7: Ambulation	131
Chapter 8: Range of Motion & Occupational Therapy	134
Chapter 9: But First Let Me Brief You	138
Chapter 10: Checks and Changes	141
Chapter 11: To The Toilet!	151
Chapter 12: Oops… There's Poo!	158
Chapter 13: Baths	171
Chapter 14: Showers	182
Chapter 15: Dressing and Undressing	190
Chapter 16: Getting Through the Day (Morn thru Night)	195
Chapter 17: Let's Get Out of Here!	201
Chapter 18: Outside Agencies and What They Do	206
Chapter 19: Hospice	213
Chapter 20: When It's All Over	229
FRUIT for Thought	235
TIPS to Remember	239
Want to go Pro?	245
In Closing	246

Introduction

Everyone will, sometime in their life, be in a caregiving situation. Whether you are giving care or receiving it, I promise!

This book is my way of helping.

In this new chapter of your life, you will need more linens. Always clean when you first put them on, only to take them off dirty.

Soiled Linens come in all shapes and sizes and may smell bizarre. However, all of them have two things in common.

1. They're covered in poo (physically and metaphorically speaking)

2. And like washcloths. They're GOLD in caregiving and hard to find.

This is You.

No, disrespect.

I think you are probably knee-deep in some metaphorical poo and if you bought this book, you are dealing with physical poo and need help. But, to the Loved One you are caring for, YOU are GOLD and hard to find.

It is okay for you to seek out help because you only want what is best.

Created by a professional with the patient and family in mind, this material holds knowledge in; caregiving, hands-on experience and information passed on by others throughout the years.

The sole purpose of Soiled Linens & Loved Ones is to support you (the Caregiver) in the act of physically caring for your Loved One. You will receive comprehensive guidelines, standard and alternative techniques to see you through your days to come. The use of this knowledge will best fit your completion of process and if possible, is manageable on the wallet.

Trials and tribulations are expected and yes, you CAN and WILL make mistakes. My goal is to help guide you through your unique circumstance, and where I found even more help is through experimentation.

Let's learn from my mistakes, shall we?

Juggling work and maybe a few little munchkins is challenging, let alone adding personal care for another to this list. Shout out to all the parents out there! You ROCK! I know those kids can be much faster than us most often.

To be a full-time caregiver is emotionally strenuous and physically demanding. Especially with someone you knew before and now, they're not the same.

Twenty-four hours a day/ seven days a week of non-stop caregiving is a doozy.

I call this "the sheets" and since you are going through it now, guess what?

You are not the only one who has "the sheets," so find a family member or friend who also has "the sheets" and become support for each other.

In order for you to succeed, you'll need to believe in yourself.

Don't worry, I got you!

Now find some friends.

Again, this book is about "Active Daily Living" care for your Loved One. I am TRYING to reach the people who probably can't afford the extra help or feel it's morally right to do the grunt work themselves.

GRUNT WORK = Everything one is obligated to do for oneself. AKA, the things everyone does for themselves on autopilot.

This is also the job title of all major multitaskers.

I should know.

You are in charge of the basic needs of your Loved One. It's only fair that you learn this from a professional "Grunt Worker" and CNA (Certified Nurse Assistant) also known as a professional caregiver.

Please don't take away from the grunt.

It's the most important part.

It's what allows people to keep their dignity in any condition they have. Helping people go on in life without skipping a beat, or at the least, at a slower pace, but still moving forward.

How you care for yourself can be taken for granted since it is our second nature.

Only when we lose the ability to do for ourselves will we truly understand its importance. What was once a task for autopilot is a humbling reality check for most.

To better understand "Grasp the Grunt"

- Meals (Dietary)
- Hygiene (Keeping Clean)
- Dressing (Getting Ready)
- Toileting (Using the Bathroom)
- Continence (Ability to hold their Bladder and Poo)
- Ambulation (Mobility)
- Activities (Stimulation)

The list goes on; however, it's THESE little things that make YOUR world go round.

Throughout these sections and chapters, you will find I have dropped FRUIT leaving important thoughts and tips to help you along the way.

Depending on your many titles concerning your Loved One and everything else you are involved in…

I CAN'T STRESS THIS ENOUGH…

You could need assistance.

Make the right decision and get some help, at least for your Loved One. Talking to your medical professional about "Support" will provide you with some insight into therapy or social groups relating to the issues at hand.

Two things stand above all that is the basis of this book; to treat others how you want to be treated and the APE Method.

Aware – Ask what the problem/issue is and accept what needs to be done.

Prepared - Prioritize your plan and follow each step with the best possible outcomes. To perform efficiently, practice a run-through with yourself in their condition before you proceed. Play the patient.

Evolving - Eliminate each step in the task list and excel with the experience gained. It helps you perform better the next time this task arises. It becomes easier the more you do it.

APE is the acronym to solve all problems or tasks you will encounter and need to overcome in your personal and professional life.

*FRUIT: Accept what is, practice what you preach, and evolve with experience. This is the key to a happy existence.

Write that down.

Following the APE method will prevent any unnecessary issues.

Injury is not the way to go, so no straying away from that, please! This will also give you visual stimulation and the rawest case scenarios.

PLEASE UNDERSTAND

I want you to know that what may work for one person may not work for another. So, work with what you have and do what you can for the best comfort of your Loved One while maintaining a clean, dry, and safe environment.

No, I'm not anal-retentive.

I've just realized that you can do caregiving securely, efficiently, quickly and cleanly without breaking your back.

A sense of responsibility is needed when doing this job because you are in charge and should any problems occur, I want you to prepare to go down with that ship.

So, make it happen, Captain!

*The more practice you have, the better you'll master it.

Ok, Grasshopper? Now try to take the pebble from my hand.

Congratulations! You have passed the most important thing to learn to provide exceptional care.

***FRUIT: The core ingredient of bedside manner is "having an interest in others without personal benefit."**

This is the crucial root of all bedside manners and providing exceptional care for your Loved One.

There are many questions people ask me when I am giving care. This is where I will answer these to provide you with a better understanding of where I am and how I have come to be here.

I am a seasoned CNA (Certified Nursing Assistant) working for hospice. My journey started at the age of thirteen helping my parents with a family friend, though professionally, I started at eighteen.

Throughout those years, I have learned lessons more than once and some more than others, many more times than one would like to brag about.

Whether you are close to someone or not, you will inevitably get close to the people you care for, building a bond and not knowing it.

All my lessons have bettered me as a caregiver during those bonding moments. I call them the Human checklist.

***FRUIT: All lessons you go through may be the same. However, one degree of difference between them makes a different lesson altogether.**

The definition of insanity is doing the same thing repeatedly and expecting a different result.

After graduating high school, Bunga (my grandmother) took me to find a job and connected me with a home-care staffing agency.

I want to touch on Bunga. As a retired maid, she has the work ethic, compassion and problem-solving role I base my profession on. She is a "No Nonsense" woman who lives true to her word. Bunga and Benny, my philosophical grandfather, who writes letters on human ethics and guidance to everyone in the family, are my second set of teachers besides my parents.

My father showed me how to care for myself, including how to survive on and off the grid. My mother, who ran a heating and air-conditioning store, showed me how to care and connect for others, instilling my sense of multitasking.

I became a PCA (Personal Care Attendant) and worked privately as a live-in caregiver for a well-off woman. It was the first time I lived away from my family doing live-in caregiving jobs in addition to other odd jobs crossing my path thereafter. I then decided to do more for myself and became a CNA who worked in a facility or two…or three.

It's there where a Hospice Aide named Yolanda (RIP) helped me with a patient and told me about hospice. I saw a chance at a change of scenery so I applied where she worked—two different ends of the spectrum.

Though I had already dealt with the death of a family member, friend and patient, it was different dealing with someone in their own home. A stranger is at the most vulnerable stage in their lives and they die in your hands. My first death while working in hospice was a man named Andrew.

I met a man who knew he was going to die. So many questions on what he was feeling at the time. He was the most pleasant man you could meet. Always ready for a shower and eager to watch the women as they strolled by. He helped me understand expectation in its better form.

A woman who hit me in my core and made me break down for the first time was named Kathrine. She lived in a facility, had no children and her only sister never came to see her. I watched this woman waste away, alone and yet was still able to smile for me. When she died, I did the necessary postmortem care, got into my car to get on the road to my next patient and burst into tears. She died with no one. I learned genuine sympathy that day.

Most recently, I couldn't tell you because there are so many and the days run into each other.

The one that hurt the most was my mother.

I was there with Bunga (her mother) when she passed. Trying to be quiet and unable to sleep, we folded clothes beside her bed. I looked at her every time she made a change in noise. Nothing prepares you for that moment, not even being a Hospice CNA.

She died at 5:51:56 AM.

I died at 5:51:56 AM.

I genuinely empathize with people who lost a parent. The world suddenly feels bigger. You are a child again, forever lost from the safest guide.

Losing a Loved One, period.

If you ask me, "Does it get easier?" No, I don't think the emotional factor changes. It all hurts, but you cry less as you see it more. You can call it "hardening," but the emotion inside never dwindles. Boy, if I had a dollar every time I was told, "I couldn't do your job."

It took me a long time to learn how to separate my work life from my home life because of how involved you are with others. Curiosity is in everyone's human nature. So, you end up swapping stories and the next thing you know, you're thinking about them while on vacation.

My parents nurtured my ability to grow as a person and without them, I wouldn't be me. But going through each of these lessons made me into the caregiver I am now and the woman I've become.

As we go through life, a critical thing for you and me is accepting what "IS" and the things you can't change. Once we are able to accept life for what it is, learn from it, our fears and regrets will dwindle, giving you a chance to focus on a better YOU.

***FRUIT: Remember, time heals what reason cannot. Your mind needs a reason and your heart needs time.**

My true happiness was fulfilled when I met and married the love of my life. Receiving me with my broken heart and all my faults, I was accepted as "me for me" and my wounds were mended. Replenished with all that I could ever need and want for my soul, I will enjoy growing old with you for the rest of my life. I love you, "Babar." Kisses from your "Farfar."

I could go on about me, but for now, there is a lot of poo to cover, so let's get this show on the road.

You are on a NEED-to-know basis and THIS you NEED to KNOW!

At some point, everyone will receive a call that changes their life.

One day that call will drop your heart to the floor.

Someone you love is in the hospital. Being there for them is essential because you will advocate for them when they cannot do so.

It is sad to say when anyone is in the hospital and has no outside support; sometimes the "Get Over" type of professional will care the bare minimum for one person while giving extra care to the family audience in the next room.

Now professionals are NOT ALL like that. Most of them are there because they care. But everywhere you go has a few "Get Overs," whether we know it or not.

Our goal as a human is to take care of one another but try to stay clear of the "Get Overs." So please be an "Advocate."

The Advocate

Imagine an elderly figure going to the hospital unresponsive. The hospital has now taken Medical Power of Attorney (POA) and will do everything possible to sustain life.

Maybe this elderly figure didn't want artificial nutrition and wanted to die naturally. Perhaps they have had their best years and didn't want to be where they are left now, to spend the rest of their days struggling due to hospital intervention.

If they could have, they would have assigned someone to speak on their behalf and their wishes would have been better met. Normally, this would be next of kin.

Before a doctor will tell you what's wrong, they will ask your Loved One for permission to speak with YOU about THEIR diagnosis. Here is where POA papers come in handy.

These POA papers are split into two parts: Financial and Medical. If your Loved One is unresponsive and you don't have these papers, doctors will do what they see fit. The court process will take so long that some patients may still be under doctor's orders until the patient passes away. Be sure to figure out your situation with your Loved One beforehand and make it work.

Because this is not my field, I recommend speaking to the social worker of the hospital or facility where your Loved One is located.

Second Opinion - If you do not accept the diagnosis, I recommend getting a second opinion. I always feel that you NEED to GET A SECOND OPINION. Confirmation is vital because sometimes things do get misdiagnosed. You just want to make sure you are not one of those people getting a misdiagnosis.

My Personal Opinion - When seeking a second opinion, leave the first diagnosis at the door. Don't go to the second doctor's office putting the diagnosis in their head, rather just let them know you're there for a second opinion and want their conclusion. Doctors are on the hunt to be the right doctor.

Opinion Three - Looking nearby if that doctor gives you a different answer.

Abuse

It is essential to know what abuse is so please look up caregiver rights as well as the rights of your Loved One. Abuse will NOT be ignored nor should it be tolerated. And keep in mind, abuse comes in all forms, not just physical.

- Physical – Physical contact causing pain to another.
- Mental and Emotional – Causing someone pain internally, verbally.
- Sexual – Physical contact that is not consented to and is done against their will.
- Neglect – Abandon, ignore, refusing to provide needed care.
- Financial – Extortion happens all the time and it is sad to say but even family members of the Loved One are capable of these heinous crimes.

Neglect is the biggest among caregiving in homes proceeded by mental abuse. The two that are most hidden are extortion and sexual abuse. They are all morally wrong and need to be watched out for. I'm sorry to say even places you think look good from the outside may have secrets.

Bring those secrets to the light if you find out about them.

None of these are okay and if you feel you could do any of these, please step away and relinquish your rights as a caregiver. The risks of continuing will harm your Loved One and may result in jail time for you.

But, if you are the caregiver being abused by your Loved One, this is not okay either. You are not a punching bag. Know you have rights just like your Loved Ones. It goes both ways.

Chapter 1: Getting To Know What You And Your Loved One Wants and Needs

This world we are in is challenging in today's times.

You are going to add another Loved One to your tribe (personal world) and you are going to need a few tools and "noggin nuggets" to conquer it all. First comes the noggin nuggets and the checklist (tools).

***FRUIT: Love is good; if you work through love a peaceful journey will surely be your path.**

First, know what you are dealing with!

Research

Research your Loved One's condition and the extent of your involvement and ask yourself one question.

Am I able to do this?

If you feel you are capable and want to continue, you need to gather the medical backstory and information of your Loved One so you may relay it to the professionals on their behalf.

***FRUIT: Whether you think you can or you can't, you're right. Your confidence is only as strong as your will.**

If you feel you cannot take on their struggles as well as yours at least help them find the right people to contact. Call their insurance (in your Loved One's presence) and find outsourced help to continue their assistance.

Please keep, read, and use this book for comparison to the care others give, with your Loved One in mind first and foremost.

But if you are ready, yell, BRING IT ON!!!

The Promise

The pledge of giving your BEST in care for others is your Promise to your Loved One.

Step 1: Sit with your Loved One, hold their hands, and look them in the eyes.

Step 2: Let them know, first and foremost, why you are helping them and then promise what you will and will not do.

Step 3: Recite this promise.

My Promise

I for you and you for me,

I promise nowhere else I'd be.

When caring for you, I put myself aside,

Leaving you comfortable with dignity and pride.

Through thick and thin, I will be heaven-sent.

To advocate for you and never resent.

I promise to listen and be gentle and kind.

To show the most compassion anyone can find,

For you are human and so am I.

So, treat me as you and I will treat you as I.

Stick to it. Sticking to things is hard, but I know you can do it. Ultimately, you will feel blessed that God gave you this opportunity to be important because you are.

I wish I could have told my mom this before she was gone.

She is the reason I wrote this book.

Check for programs pertaining to the conditions of your Loved One because you may qualify for more support for them. Learn about your Loved One's insurance and medical endeavors and what is or isn't covered by their insurance. After this, adjust the insurance to qualify for their needs and wants.

Let's check on physical well-being.

Physical Assessment of the Body

Checking their body inside the hospital will let you know if any wounds are visible and need to be addressed before you take them home.

Physically assess your Loved One again when they get home so you know if there is anything that you didn't already find in the hospital. Check the body all over unclothed. I don't mean strip them down to birthday suits, but looking at their skin frequently will prevent unnecessary wounds.

Reddened areas aren't to be taken lightly. The skin is our body's largest organ and the visual indicator of something wrong.

Next would be the eyes and then check inside the mouth. Pee and Poo is also an indicator, but I'll touch on that later. The most common red area, not seen very often, but can get nasty, is the tail bone (Coccyx), so be on the lookout.

If they come home with sores, wounds, bumps and/or bruises, keeping these tended to and monitored until resolved is crucial to the healing process (See Wound Care).

After leaving the hospital, they will follow up with a home care nurse and CNA for a month or two after arriving home. They will no longer continue after that and if you need more assistance, I recommend looking into home health agencies (See Chapter 18 Outside Agencies and What they Do).

Emergency Watch For Symptoms

Pay attention to any emergency symptoms that need attending to and monitored until resolved or accommodated for easy Daily Living. Should these particular symptoms arise, they should not be ignored.

1. Chest pain and shortness of breath can be a heart attack

2. Weakness and numbness can be a stroke or an initial warning for a more significant stroke.

3. 102 Temperature that won't break can mean numerous things

4. Unbearable headache that won't subside. Possible brain swelling. I'm talking, "I'm going to die type pain!!!!"

5. Blindness can mean neurological issues and more. An ophthalmologist can make sure their eyes are ok. You don't want their retina to detach and leave them permanently blind.

6. Acute pain that debilitates your Loved One to the fetal position can be kidney stones, kidney infection, or something worse.

7. Swelling of the leg and feeling hot to the touch may be a sign of a blood clot ready to travel to the heart.

There are many things to look for, but anything out of the normal that won't subside is debilitating and needs assistance beyond your control.

Keeping up with any symptoms may prevent or help with any other conditions your Loved One may have acquired.

Treatments

Symptoms from their condition are treated with medication, dietary and physical regiments, and a lot of praying.

Please follow the doctor's directions before, during and after and make sure you listen! I've seen the aftermaths of not following the treatment "plans and procedures." It's NOT pretty.

Monitor and Document all change in activity and reactions with length of time taken to subside. Adjust to the individual as you go. If you are unable to control with medications and other treatments provided, seek medical attention.

Precautions

Read all information given about conditions and medications so you are prepared for any precautions to take should you notice any side effects.

If you do, go to the ER Stat (Immediately)!

Keep medical devices and medications available and research all medical hacks to help subside any symptoms if your treatments aren't available for future problematic moments.

Find possible Programs you qualify for to help support your specific situation. Research more about the condition(s) your Loved One has to better understand where their heads are and what they are going through.

Give them what they wish for and have it laid out. These Loved Ones are adults and pretty much know what they want in store for their future. Allow them to make that decision (IF they can do so).

Danger and Risks

You need to be able to resolve anything in a time-sensitive manner. You are racing time before there is nothing more you can do and you have to seek professional medical attention.

Danger happens when risks or no action is taken.

Thoroughly think it out promptly and ensure you are positive about whatever risk you are willing to take. The real dangers lie in the consequential outcome.

***FRUIT: When it's done it's done, no turning back. So, calculate the risk and please be at peace with the outcome. Good luck.**

Learn all safety precautions before doing any task that involves you moving your Loved One. Again, not every person needs the same care, if care is for more than one, they may not want it done the same way. You must listen to them and see what it is they want as each person may explain it differently. However, when the task is done, make sure the end result is the same: Completed and Safe.

In order to do so, you need some Main Essentials (Tools).

Main Essentials (Tools)

Like Batman, you need your weapons. These are things you need to tackle your battles with victory. I've split it into two main essentials, one for you and one for your Loved One.

<u>**For you**</u>:

Support = A Sidekick

Records = A Journal

Risk and Side effects = What causes your stress

Policy = Human Checklist

Who's Your Sidekick?

Every superhero out there (like you) needs a sidekick. i.e., Batman and Robin. A co-caregiver. Someone to take over while you are absent and can help as if you were there. They need to know what you know and you'll work together as one. You need a break periodically and your sidekick should cover you. Take that break!

Or you WILL break yourself!

And don't forget to appreciate them. They are going through what you are, so please don't discredit them from what they deserve.

For my family, my sister and I have established our roles for my father. She is in the same city as him and now helps care for his needs. My brother will watch over my grandparents. While later down the road, I will be in charge of my father's care, allowing him to go the way he would like medically and naturally AKA the well-being or dying process. I will do the same for my grandparents and siblings unless I go first.

I'm a proud sidekick!

Journal

Creating a journal will assist in the record of your Loved One's life and keep their physicians informed accurately. Highlighters are a big way for you to see all you need to in one chronological order. Color chart example below will program your eyes to process information faster while relaying it to the professional. This also gives you more time to cover all other inquiries within that visit. Color code to your desire.

- **Meds** Yellow
- **Meals** Blue
- **Poop &Pee** Brown
- **Showers** Purple
- **Injuries** Red
- **Mental State** Green

Shorthand helps write faster. There are some commonly used words in the medical field you may want to familiarize yourself with to help when going to doctor appointments. These records will help them skim through your Loved One's life.

- **BM = Bowel Movement**
- **XS S M L XL = Sizes**
- **BID = twice a day**
- **Q = Every**
- **PER = Says _____ ex: Says Who? PER me!**
- **X = how many times ex: 3x daily**

Anything other than these, I usually take out all the vowels. When you dedicate your writing style, be consistent with it.

Once, I tried to write fast and correct, but my speed was faster than my correction. You may not have the same issue considering I was caring for more than one person, regardless be sure to maintain consistency.

Only write important things. Nobody needs to know when your Loved One farted (depending on the situation), but they may need to know when they had a Bowel Movement (BM).

You Time, aka Risks and Side Effects

It is necessary to always remember to take care of yourself so you may care for another. If something happens to you because you weren't there, you'll feel the ultimate lowest.

So, utilizing your sidekick and getting six to eight hours of sleep is imperative.

Don't forget to feed yourself too.

Plan alone time. I don't care how you spend time behind closed doors, just as long as they are closed and there is space for you to escape. (Kidding)

Your Stress Causes

1. **Anxiety**
    a. Feelings of anxiety weighs on your body and mind like a drenched winter coat. Please search for ways to treat your anxiety.
    b. The most common way to help calm yourself is good meditation and breathing. Take time to breathe.

2. **Forgetfulness**
    a. Forgetfulness may not affect you until you forget something that will turn your life upside down.
    b. Posting notes in places I frequent has helped me tremendously. Other than that, I can't help you here. Lapse in memory is going to happen therefore, be creative.

3. **Extra Medical Conditions**
    a. Scheduling and keeping up with your doctor appointments will maintain your health and well-being.

4. **Issues you may have that can't be explained**
    a. Unexplainable issues symbolize nothing seems to be going right and the universe is on its own wavelength. When it rains, it pours.

How to Deplete Your Stress

1. The "You Time" should be sufficient, but some people may need more time than others so plan accordingly.
2. Some form of therapy will help you talk out your struggles.
3. Time out for yourself is so vital; go shopping, do hobbies, or even feed the birds. Caregiver Burnout is a big cause for you to take a break from all things and make time for YOURSELF to spend time with YOURSELF. Remember, it is ok to say no and take a nap. Try good exercise and a nutritional diet. But remember, there is a thin line between saying no and straight-up neglect.

Human Checklist

The lessons I've learned for myself to get through and then lessons dealing with others.

1. I understand the most vital thing to keep you going through life with dignity is to take full ***RESPONSIBILITY*** for your decisions, actions and words. Your decisions will determine your actions and your words hold so much power to manifest what you want or even what you don't. This is pertinent to understand you are responsible for everything pertaining to you. When you take on the responsibility of another, you are responsible from a legal standpoint for the livelihood of your Loved One. Own it and watch yourself.

2. ***SELF-PRESERVATION*** is vital. I don't mean to be selfish, but if you do not take care of yourself and consider yourself, you will put yourself in a sticky situation you didn't prepare for. If you don't take care, how can you possibly take care of another? It's okay to say no without neglect, but keep in mind the thin line between. Enough about you.

3. Growing up, I've learned that I don't know everything and don't know what others need, want, or have gone through. As much as I think I know, I have been proven wrong on many occasions. One of the biggest of mine is history and politics, which not having enough knowledge about the subjects, makes me feel I don't have the right to talk about them. To assume makes an ASS out of U and ME. So, please ***LISTEN*** to yourself, your Loved One and others.

4. I look at ***SYMPATHY and EMPATHY*** and ensure I know the difference and correctly respond when it's due. When thinking of others, have sympathy for shoes you haven't walked in and have empathy for those you have. I see people who induce these feelings and will make me try to do something good for them. It is where compassion originates from.

5. My mother taught me to treat others how I want to be treated, with kindness. Now, this is **_COMPASSION_** for me.

6. **_HUMILITY_** keeps my pride in check. When you are there to help others and treat them as if your feelings are above them, you better check your pride. As you walk down the street one day and see another in worse shape than you are, please remember you are always one step away from falling down a flight of stairs. Stay Humble. But on the other hand, don't take away from **_PRIDE_** in what you do because if you don't take pride, you'll only do as good as your pride allows you. We may come to waste away, but our **_DIGNITY_** never dies. Let humiliation die instead by letting them keep their dignity.

7. Having **_PATIENCE_** teaches you how to wait patiently until you are needed. It teaches how to slow down your thinking brain to clear and reset. I also notice that when I rush, I take longer than I expected. You'll be surprised if you slow down how fast things come to you. Good things come to those who wait.

8. Life is hard and not only do you protect yourself, but you also have to be an **_ADVOCATE_** for others regardless of the situation. If you see something, you should say something. You advocate for the victim from a moral standpoint until the correct professional can take over—someone equipped to advocate for them morally. If you find any abuse, you must advocate immediately and get help.

9. Understand the **_SIGNIFICANCE_** of what you are doing and consider its possible outcome. Make sure you know what is more important than others and then decide on the outweighing of all factors. It will help you

put your tasks in order of severity. You are vital and without you, your Loved One couldn't thrive.

10. **_CONSISTENCY_** is key for your Loved One to have a daily routine and assurance in life in general. They will have more confidence in using their strength, knowing they can consistently rely on your presence and ensure they are always okay. The consistency automatically lets them know the tasks at hand and may even jump-start them to get completed. Even if you can't be there, have others help. Remember, it's always nice to see the same faces.

11. Learn to be **_GENTLE_**. People are frail physically and, at times, vulnerable in many ways. It's easier to learn how to be strong, but way harder to be gentle. Always ask about the level of tenderness so you can adjust to their comfortability. You can come off harsh and don't mean it, but don't fret, just adjust.

12. Sometimes things happen that cannot be reversed and you will feel a certain amount of **_REGRET_**. No one can tell you how or how not to feel, but it doesn't make this regret disappear, regardless of how hard you try. Attempt to take it one day at a time because time heals what reason cannot. This is easier said than done, but nevertheless, you'll learn how to **_FORGIVE_** yourself. It is hard, but remember you are perfect in your own imperfect way.

13. **_GRIEF_** is the moment you are going through your deepest sorrows and has no average length of stay for each stage. Some levels of grief are harder depending on the sorrows. Here is the order of the seven stages of grief for every situation.

This is the standard order though I have seen others experience them in different sequences:

1. Shock
2. Denial
3. Anger
4. Bargaining
5. Depression
6. Testing
7. Acceptance

***FRUIT: Have sympathy for others for you may be there one day, then we'd be talking about empathy.**

***FRUIT: It's not what you have. It is what you feel when you enjoy what you have. <u>*HAPPINESS*</u> also equals <u>*JOY*</u>. But understand happiness comes when you find joy in your life. The little joys add up to happiness.**

I would explain how I got to these lessons, but I'll save that for a different book entirely. These core lessons of mine were taught to me by my most dear parents and grandparents. My spouse, siblings, cousins, and friends also helped me through it, riding by my side. We're all here on earth, meant to learn and change from the lessons learned to elevate our self-worth. I've gone through these lessons repeatedly, but have always been in a different situation. Be open to receiving, evolving and moving on to other tools.

For Your Loved One

Main Essentials and Problem Reliever Checklists

It will be easier for you if you have everything you need and are going to use, handy or close by. But it's even better for your Loved One, so they can be more independent and help them not rely on others as much. Some people prefer to do more for themselves.

I hope you're that lucky. But for the rest of us who don't have that luxury, it's good to have an easy setup to Grab n' Continue.

Main Essentials Checklist

Requested periodically but often enough to keep nearby.

1. **Pillows** - You can never have too many, four minimum. I will speak about how to place them in repositioning later, but for the best comfort, I recommend four.

2. **Blankets** - (As many as they wish) two minimum. Sometimes people may run hot and ask why they have extra, but you never know.

3. **Bedside Table** - (Comes in handy, TRUST!) Some fill it with a bunch of stuff they don't need. Get a second bedside table.

4. **A Cooling and Heating source**. - Fan and heater, keep them comfortable and temped, or tempers fly high. Some people like natural cooling, so maybe those blankets come in handy for you instead.

5. **T.V.** - No one wants to look at a wall all day if they're with it. Please remember that a remote is portable; consider tying it to the bed. My lady Kathryn came up with that conclusion when she kept losing her remote and I kept finding it under her bottom or on the floor.

6. <u>**Music source**</u>. - A lot of people prefer to hear a melody they know verses random people's voices on T.V. Sometimes, it sounds like just a bunch of noise. I play a lot of music from my personal phone while helping my people with baths or showers. It takes a lot of attention from them being naked in front of a stranger, let alone the opposite sex. Some men live for that and then they meet James with the tattoos. Thanks, James, You're one awesome possum. He was also able to calm the crazy ladies. They acted like perfect angels in his presence. They think he's hot.

7. <u>**Tissue**</u> - There isn't a soul I took care of that didn't keep asking for a tissue. Some people like to stuff them in their sleeves, so check before throwing them in the wash. Now, this is more so with women, but you have those men constantly spitting or blowing their noses, so check all their pockets.

8. <u>**Trash Can**</u> near the bed - self-explanatory. Need I say more.

9. <u>**Call Bell**</u> - Anything that makes a distinct noise. The button doorbells are popularly used, but I've seen a call bell as cheap as a bulb horn. ANYTHING that makes a distinct noise will work.

10. <u>**Constant Drink and Snack**</u> - Straws are handy for many reasons. Having a Constant cold drink and refreshed when needed is comforting to know they won't die of dehydration in this bed. *If* your Loved One cannot do it for themselves, you need to ask them if they are thirsty and to offer often. Consider snacks that don't get old too fast.

11. <u>**Hobbies**</u> – anything for your Loved One to pass the time during recovery.

BOOM!

All other necessities will be further explained with specific tasks at hand.

Know your most common problems & solutions

The world isn't perfect and problems can arise. You name it, it can probably happen to you.

You are a freaking unicorn you!

Solving the world's problems isn't your job—just the problems of you and your Loved One.

You're the captain.

Make it happen!

Problems will often occur and a few are relatively easy to solve. Others are; however, not that easy. You need to learn a few things before approaching the situation.

You need to know about communication.

Communication

Communication between you and your Loved One is the most straightforward problem-solving task. You need to be open and honest with each other, so no one has any harsh feelings if a problem arises.

Recognize there are additional "Magic Words" besides "Please" and "Thank You." "Help Me Understand" are good "Magic Words."

Patience

Know it well.

You must show that you are there for them and them only. Trying your best, you must do this and only this to complete everything satisfactorily to not just your satisfaction, but theirs as well! Make them see you are trying to help them, not hinder them.

Ways to communicate are essential! If speaking is hard, come up with your own yes/no sign language. Letting other people know the yes/no language will communicate better and may release unnecessary stress. I see a lady that answers Yes/No questions with a thumbs up or down.

For people who want to communicate more complexly, a word board fit to your Loved One would help. Phones are more equipped than before. I helped a lady with a word board with the alphabet and a certain amount of choice words and emotions to express herself more precisely.

Find what works.

Talk about the Problem – Most likely, it is something they can tell you and probably can be solved immediately. In time, though, it can be harder to find a resolution.

Discomfort

If they are unresponsive, you may need to watch their body language and facial grimacing closely. Please don't think they can't hear you in their physical state as your comments may be brought up later.

Awkward.

The process of elimination, to find the proper comfort for an unresponsive Loved One, is sometimes lengthy but, at most times, is just a move of a sheet. Wrinkles can hurt after a while.

Have a problem?

Let's relieve it. Check these questions first.

Problem RELIEVER Checklist

1. See if they are positioned right (See "Save a Member Checklist" in Mantra Section for Repositioning)

2. Are the sheets flat and wrinkle-free behind them?

3. Are they too hot or cold?

4. Do they need to use the restroom or do they need to be cleaned up after doing so?

5. Are they thirsty?

6. Are they hungry?

7. Is the lighting or noise bothering them?

8. Finally, are they in pain and just need some Medication?!!!!!

I usually save the medicine for last because that will exhaust all other options so it must be pain. This prevents any unnecessary medication.

Forgetfulness and Repetitiveness

Forgetfulness is challenging to deal with, especially if you are the one going through it. I have experienced something where I forgot what I was doing and where I was going, driving around in circles, and breaking down crying. Now imagine that, but five times worse, because that may be what your Loved One is going through. Sometimes they can't snap out of it.

Empathize, repeat what they need to hear, and remember to have compassion and patience instead of looking at them as crazy. Help them remember. Sing it in a song. A melody helps retain better.

***FRUIT: Control of our minds is what we hold dear so don't hold it against others if they lose it.**

Although you may or may not deal with a change of mind, forgetfulness becomes a habit of nature and may not be something the caregiver is used to. Please don't hold it against them. Things happens It's not the end of the world if they keep asking you to repeat what you said. You will repeat yourself with the outside world anyway, so what makes this different?

Brain Farts

Brain farts are common among caregivers.

There is so much to remember that sometimes you forget tasks needed to get done. It sucks when these tasks are essential.

But this happens.

If you have brain farts more than usual, maybe you should take a break. Have your sidekick come in and help. When your brain farts too much, it's your brain that needs a break even though you feel FINE = F'd up, Insecure, Neurotic and Emotional.

To help with this, a calendar to write appointments, events and deadlines will ease that noggin from gassing up the place. Writing things down or setting multiple alarms with notes helps me. Alexa is good at waking me up but bad at listening sometimes.

You will have to make changes to the plan of care you provide as you go along. Just like how your Loved One's condition changes so will your care plan. The more changes, the more care needed and more notes posted. Like Laverne & Shirley, they go hand-in-hand.

Learning the best schedule for you both

Both you and your Loved One may be on two different schedules, so it is important to compromise on times, including personal.

If you two are constantly with each other, at some point, you won't like each other for the moment. So, make sure there is something they still enjoy or a new hobby while you are doing your own thing. Maybe you will share a common interest enough to enjoy hobbies together, but make sure you have time to yourself as well as others.

Set up a scheduled time for all essential things needed daily and stick to the plan. Consistency is key for a productive day even if you are not doing anything. Now you may have to repeat yourself, so make a song of it.

Should all the needs be met and your Loved One is still unsettled or unhappy, talk to them more. Dig deep into their feelings and try to see what's on their mind. Try to understand them better. Sometimes people need to talk to another person to feel human.

This is called helping their soul.

Be cautious that some people may want to be left alone, you don't want to be overbearing, do you? Some people call this smothering.

Chapter 2: Universal Precautions - They're Coming Home!

Huh? Whaaat?!

Universal Precautions = Everything Prepared for.

It Means to Prepare for ANYTHING related to YOUR situation! I want you to be prepared for anything that comes your way and no, I don't know everything, but I will tell you as much as I can.

For all occasions, you should be quick thinking, fast acting, and accountable while still keeping your cool. Remember all your tasks and remind yourself of the universal precautions needed for a safe result.

*FRUIT: Making haste makes waste.

You know how you catch every light when you rush to get somewhere? It's Murphy's law in action. I'm not telling you to rush through without thinking and I'm not telling you to go sloth mode, either. I just want you to think things through before you make a decision or act too fast.

Be prepared for any altering obstacles from your wanted outcome. To do this, you want to have a great starting route. For example, if attempting to give a Loved One a shower, the process may go something like this:

1. Plan A: get things ready to give a shower
2. Plan B: if your Loved One gets woozy, you would already have a shower chair available within reach and extra towels in the dryer

3.   Meanwhile, while assisting your Loved One, begin thinking of a Plan C just in case. This may be having your sidekick on standby to grab anything extra you may need. This way, you don't have to leave your Loved One by themselves or it may be as simple as having a wheelchair ready if needed.

4.   If you stop along the route, be sure to leave your Loved One in a safe place to fix any altering task. If safety is an issue, leave the task and take care of the safety issue until you can try again and your Loved One is willing. This may be something like forgetting an item you initially needed or a health issue arising midway through completing the shower.

You are a fish going with the flow with what works and cleaning as you go. You may have to clean up later, but don't let it sit as you may not have the oomph if you wait too long.

A.P.E. Method in an "Oh Shit" Situation

Assess. Plan. Execute

No one is perfect. And you are the best at what you do. When a solution isn't clear, step back and re-evaluate your situation. Let's reclaim the meaning of going APESHIT!

Assess & **P**lan to **E**liminate **S**ituations **H**inderingly **I**nitiating **T**urmoil

What does it mean?

One thing that needs to be A.P.E.'d the quickest is a medical emergency such as someone who is unresponsive or goes into cardiac arrest.

I can't repeat this enough for fellow caregivers; grab the chance to take a class in First Aid and Cardio Pulmonary Resuscitation (CPR). It will cover how to do CPR on an adult, child, and infant along with different ways to do the Heimlich maneuver for choking, and the procedure for seizures. The internet has the latest reviews and updated tips if classes are unavailable.

The medical field continuously revises its protocols to be faster and more efficient. Even if done correctly, the manual CPR success rate is very slim. What is most effective now are Automated External Defibrillator (AED) machines. Its purpose is used for reviving a pulse while walking you through the CPR process. It has bumped the survival rate immensely and gives a lot of confidence to people thrust into that situation.

To do CPR properly your Loved One has to be on a flat and hard surface to ensure your compressions are strong enough to reach the heart. Most people need to be slid or pushed to the floor to start CPR; however, some people are hard to move because of "dead weight" at which point you would need to find something hard and flat to substitute for a hard surface, placing it underneath their back to start chest compressions while breathing for them.

Don't forget to call 911. These things are hard to do all at once for one person. And with all the emotional stress and shock, it may draw a blank in your mind.

I recommend having an AED machine in conjunction with CPR. They are not cheap, but think about investing in one…I am. It's a scary situation to be in. Keep in mind, an AED machine will only bring back a pulse so if your Loved One has stopped breathing, you will still need to breathe for them.

Certification for First Aid and CPR is only good for two years and needs to be renewed for all the revised and updated information and techniques. So, keep up with it.

Another scary situation is fighting for your life from something you can't see. A lot of times, that's happening with germs and diseases. Contagions are enemies to your body and catching something can be prevented if you know about it.

Here are three ways you can catch something:

Transmission of Infection Precautions

These are measures observed and maintained so you may identify the type of transmission of infection and the proper procedures taken to prevent and spread infection.

It is imperative to know the transmission variants when exposed to any contagions.

1. Contact- Self-explanatory.
   a. Direct- Physical Contact to you directly from the infected
   b. Indirect- Contact between you and the infected is taking the same route, touching the same surface, area, or object.

2. Droplet- Direct and Indirect.
   a. Any fluids or secretions that come in contact with you, like blood, spit, sweat, etc. Something too heavy to be carried through the air.
   b. There is a droplet radius depending on the weight.

3. Airborne- Run for your life; I'm just kidding. That's how people act.
   a. It needs to be quarantined.
   b. Lightweight and can travel through the air at long distances.
   c. Because it needs immediate attention, consult your physician for further instructions.

Personal Protective Equipment

(PPE) is anything added to protect each individual from contamination. Usually, clean your hands with soap and water; it's best to be safe than sorry. Most common include, but are not limited to:

1. Gloves - self-explanatory
   a. Doubling up on gloves while in use can help you save time washing hands to change gloves during messy tasks.
   b. There are also glove types for allergens such as having a latex allergy

2. Masks - consists of but not limited to
   a. surgical mask just covers for droplets
   b. N95 mask for air contaminants

3. Face Shield – acts as an eye contact preventative.
   a. Goggles are also a good form of eye protectant (people don't know how hard it is to give a hot shower with goggles on and my goodness, with a face shield)

4. Booties are disposable Shoe Covers
5. Hair cap (rare in the home but possible)
6. Gowns can be cloth or disposable.
   a. The most common gowns are paper towel thin or plastic.

All these are available to the public and if you get it like that, make sure to buy in bulk. You will go through them like candy and not know it until you need it. Otherwise, be sparing when using and figure out which tasks are okay to deal with using soap and water and which needs more protection.

Hand Washing Safety Measures

Wash your hands and or sanitize when?

1. Before you start.
2. After you are done.
3. When visibly soiled. (Wash)
4. When you dig in orifices. (Wash your hands!)
5. Sanitizers work in between washes, two to three maximum for me, or you'll feel the grit on your hands.

Wear gloves during any task dealing with physical contact or touching anything infected or too personal.

If your gloves are soiled and you must go and touch a clean area or other regions, change your gloves or remove the top layer to reveal the new set. If you are dealing with a contagion, you will reduce the spread this way.

*FRUIT: If in doubt, double up when gloving up.

*FRUIT: Sanitizer is not SOAP! You can use sanitizer three uses max before you need to wash your hands.

Things happens fast and sometimes you run out of gloves.

Guess what?

Hand Washing Process

Wash your hands before and after helping with any soiling.

When you sweat, you might wipe it subconsciously. Now you have feces on your face. Okay, I understand when things happen fast and sometimes you aren't always prepared; I have that happen too. Make sure you graduate from soap and water school.

I would invest in a nail brush.

Get the antibacterial and scrub vigorously your hands, nails and all the way up to the elbows. Hitting all over and double-check these areas:

1. Between the fingers
2. The whole thumb down to the wrist
3. The back side of your hand
4. Along the pinky down to the wrist

5. Scrub brush helps, but if you're without, use your nails in the middle of the palms.

6. Tell you what, sing a song that lasts thirty seconds or longer while you scrub.

7. Rinse thoroughly

8. Dry with paper towels or a clean, dry cloth

9. Then turn the water off with a paper towel or dry cloth you used.

If you have an itch you can't ignore, use the higher part of the arm/shoulder to get it.

Environmental Precautions

Ensuring your Loved One's environment stays clean and safe will prevent your day from being interrupted by excess tasks.

Have your cleaning items put away, but easy to get to. You can never go wrong with disinfectant cleaning wipes. Wipe things down, especially wherever you or your Loved One touch frequently.

Not saying y'all are dirty, but you don't want them to catch anything and you certainly don't want to give them anything. If you are sick with a cold, you might need to use PPE.

These are the most common places touched and in dire need of disinfectant.

1. Doorknobs
2. Door Frames
3. Sink/ Handles
4. Commonly used surfaces

5. Railings
6. Toilet Handles
7. TV Remotes etc.
8. Light Switches

You get my drift. Don't forget your phone, cards and keys (used the most).

Now that you are safe inside, how do you get out?

First and foremost, safety is key and an escape plan is crucial for that.

My father instilled in me that if you enter a building, look for your exits first. If something happens beyond your control and going through the front is not an option to leave, you should always know where the alternate exits are and plan your escape safely and timely before it's too late.

Like a fire escape plan, make sure there are no obstacles in the way of your departure.

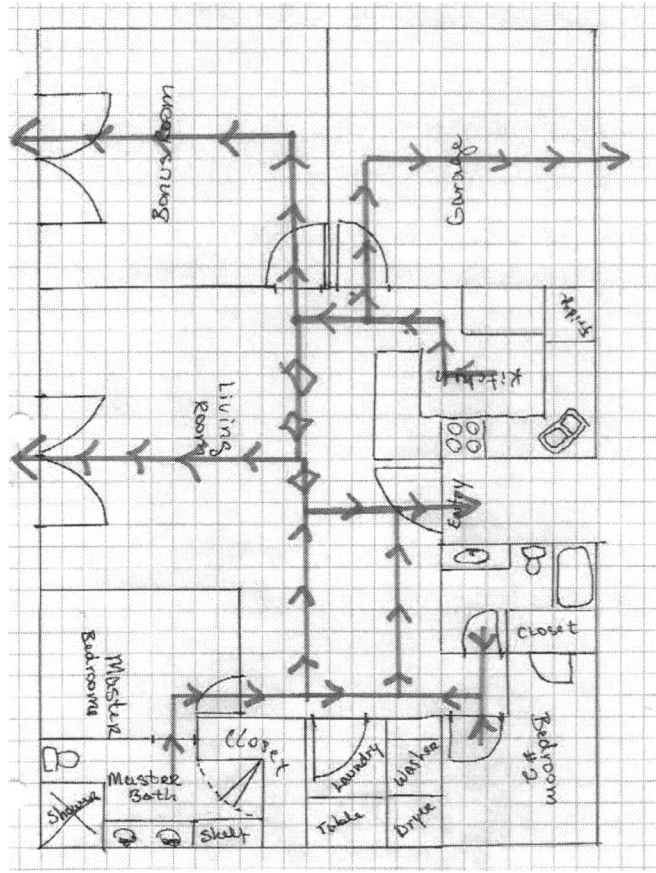

    It is vital to prepare your environment for the arrival of your Loved One and to make sure they feel safe in that environment. Don't stick them in the corner hidden away in a storage room because they will feel like a burden. Ensure they feel this room is only for them and their comfort. Burden feelings are hard to get rid of. Reassure them constantly in a loving manner that you are happy they are there with you.

Please always be aware of the scary fall precautions in this diagram, it will show you possible corners that cause injury.

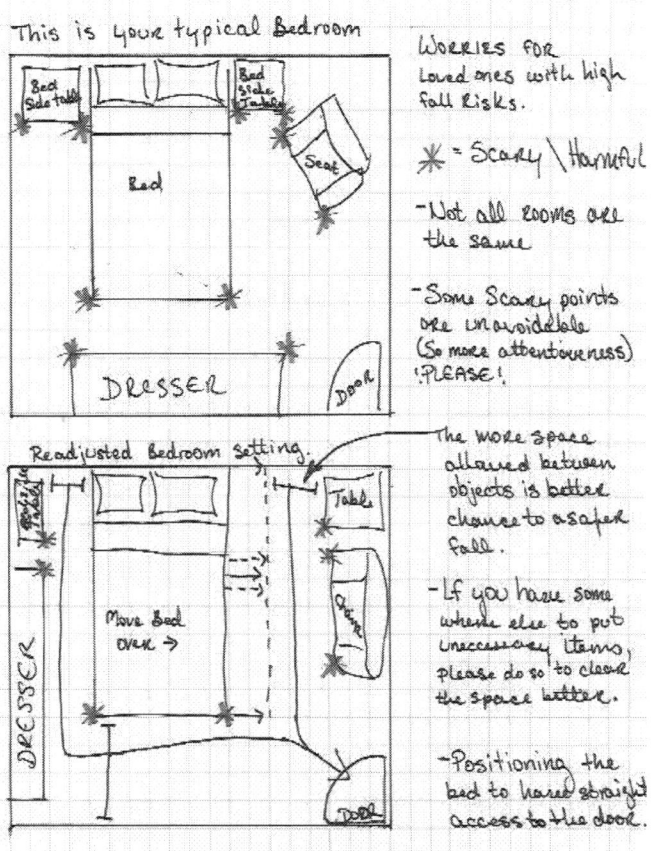

Environmental Setup

Your Loved One's room has red flags that will catch someone's eye. Any area that comes to your attention for the possible fall risk moment, whether tripping or slipping, needs brace points.

Many choices of brace points can also be a hindrance. People going down and having too many brace points to choose from may not make a decision in time before impact. Learning how to fall properly will lessen the blows taken from falling.

And one thing we may all do is tense up waiting for impact. We all must learn how to relax our bodies and turn them into wet noodles. I don't think anyone has heard of a good boat roll; our face usually stops us from doing that.

Let's Play a Game.

I want you to scan all the rooms used by your Loved One, find and flag all scary points for possible injury, and see how many you can find and then fix them. As a preventative measure, scan for any mishaps that could happen due to potential obstacles that are in the way. See if your Loved One is physically safe to be where they are and move anything sharp-edged. Should they fall, they won't fall on that.

Things that are unsafe make a plenty long list, so I'll just give a few examples. After, I want you to spot those things and others you can think of in your home.

Make it a game and hunt them all out. Put on your safety scanner goggles.

1. Anything that rolls and has locks.
   a. Make sure it is easy to manipulate and all locks are **ON** when not using or need to be stable.
2. Slippery or wet floors. Nonskid socks or skid-resistant shoes help with this common issue.
   a. Clean up any spills as soon as you are aware of them. Putting it off sets you up for hurt or guilt later.
3. Rugs and Cords etc.
   a. Pick up all loose rugs and tape down all exposed cords. If rugs are necessary, please include slide-resistant material under the rug to help prevent the problems caused by rugs.
4. Sharp corners
   a. Everyone can fall and boy, do they like to fall down by sharp corners. Heart attack city you'll live in if you don't get those corners covered with some protective material.
5. Light furniture that moves quickly and easily.

Unsteady furniture, or furniture that can move with the weight of your body, takes part in almost every fall. Your Loved One feels like they are about to fall, so they grab the furniture hoping it will hold their weight. But if it's light and has no friction under it to do that, say you are sorry now rather than later.

This is where a rug can come in a little handier for you. Just put it under the feet of the furniture, with slide-resistant material under it.

Bathroom – Needs to be dry and safe upon entering to use the restroom or shower. For the use of the toilet, please keep in mind the sharp edges and spaces with no brace point.

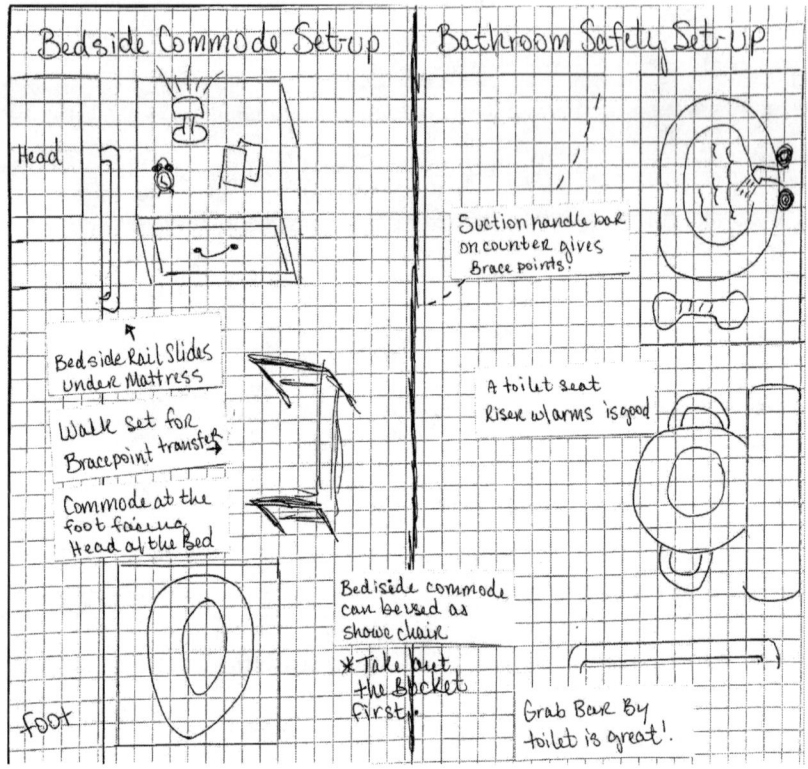

The Toilet is versatile if you have a bedside commode. You don't have to walk far.

You can never have too many handlebars for safety and brace points. Dizziness can happen anywhere and the bedroom and bathroom are the most dangerous places for it to happen.

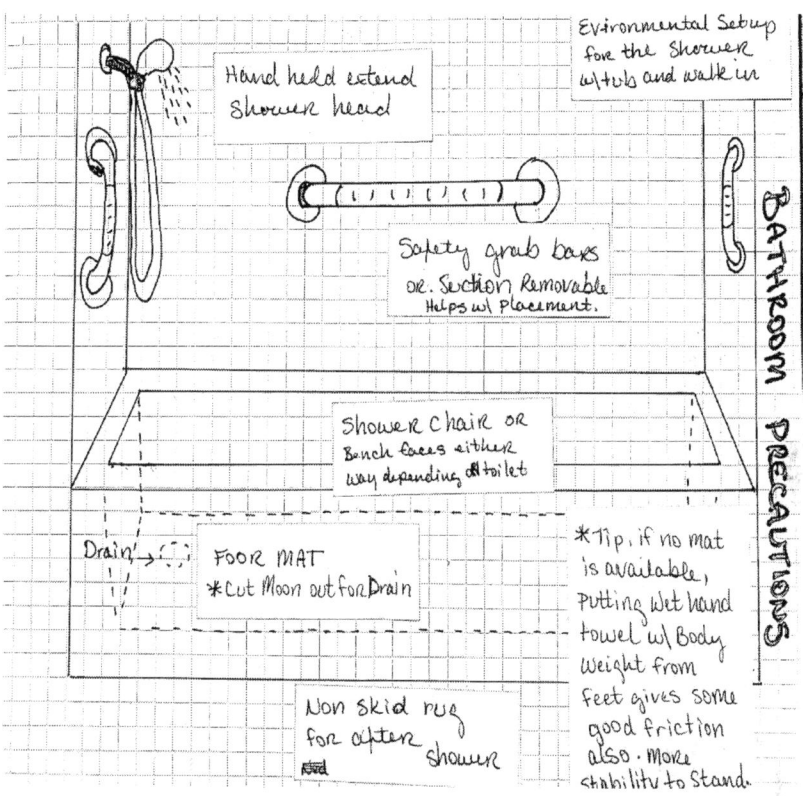

The Do's

1. Furniture placement is vital for fluid ambulation and transfers, lowering the risk factor. For high-risk Loved Ones, keeping the nightstand further away from the bed will help. It lowers the risk of your Loved One sitting up too fast, getting dizzy and falling near the nightstand, resulting in a head injury.

2. Locking all wheels of anything that rolls.

3. Remove lightweight furniture from areas that your Loved One might use to lean on or replace it with heavier ones.

4. Pick up all rugs and loose items off the floor as they are tripping hazards. Keeping pathways clear is also a good idea.

5. Having a tall shelf to put all your necessities on will keep it more organized for you. Starting at the top with dry items, going down the bottom and ending with liquids.

6. Line all cords along the walls. Try not to cross walkways, but if you have to, please tape them down. But other than that, extension cords are a plus. Power strips with surge protection is best. You don't want to start crying because your TV blew.

7. Lighting needs to be perfect. Meaning if it's dark outside, you need enough light inside to turn it into daytime. Psychologically, this also can help people who suffer from sun-downing. And you don't want a spill of some sort to happen and you can't see what you are cleaning or even if your Loved One is safe.

8. Putting a two by four wood plank between the bed and your wall will save the wall from any damage the bed may cause from constant moving of your Loved One or protruding bed parts.

The Don'ts

- Everything opposite of the list above.

Don't even think about it

1. For sure, No Smoking while oxygen is in use. It can turn into a rocket as well as a bomb. You might want to look that up.

2. No petroleum jelly-based substances are used on the face of people with oxygen assistance. Chapstick, Vaseline, etc. Very, very flammable and the face can catch fire.

3.   Never leave your Loved One in a position for disaster. Ensure they are safe, secure, and clean so there will be less of a reason to move around while you are away. If in a wheelchair, make sure the locks are engaged.

Dangers and Risks

Not paying attention to the possible dangers and risks of your Loved One's environment can cause massive destruction to your life or worse, theirs. Ask questions every time a factor in your situation changes. Example: If I leave, what can possibly happen to them and how can I avoid those disasters? Placement is key. And remember to COMPLETE every task by putting everything back in its place after you are done.

Start the process for soiled linens and throw away any trash. Procrastination can slow you down, become overwhelming, and make you resentful and not wanting to do any of it.

Know your Loved One's safety limits and acknowledge all possible dangers and risks in the situation you are dealing with. Whatever is considered a danger to try is a big "NO, NO," and things with higher risks of being dangerous is also considered NOT to do. If your Loved One is too heavy to lift from a fall, for example, it's a big "no-no" to lift on your own if you don't know the techniques. We will hit this later in the mantra section. The best bet is to get help or call the fire department.

Safety Assessment and Measures to take

Evaluate how bad the situation is that you're in and play out a decision in your mind showing you every good and bad possibility all the way to the end result, in one of these categories.

1. Safe
   a. lying on the bed,
   b. sitting in the chair, or
   c. standing braced with stability assistance of some kind (a walker, for example)
2. Unsafe
   a. On the floor (Safest of All the unsafe)
   b. On the floor bleeding
   c. On the floor bleeding and or broken
   d. Worse, not breathing and or unresponsive.
3. What things make it unsafe
   a. Chair unlocked or not secured.
   b. Bed wheels unlocked, railings down or in a high elevation.
   c. Slippery or wet floors
   d. Movable rugs or no rugs for friction, etc.

Rugs have their safe and unsafe points. If a rug is down, it should hold steady heavy objects which, in return, will hold the rug down safely. A rug with no serious contributor can be a tripping hazard and needs a non-skid underbelly, or just remove it.

Predicaments are going to happen.

No matter how hard you try, a new predicament you didn't see coming will arise. Don't worry and don't beat yourself up about it. Things happen all the time and YOU can't protect from everything. Just remember two words you are going to say a LOT.

"It's okay," I say this with love because you need to know that this is a moment in time that, too, will soon pass.

So, guess what?

It's okay, my love. Now focus.

Consider the A.P.E. Method and Assess the predicament and evaluate.

All predicaments have some path leading to worse ones. Knowing how to stay calm in these situations is crucial for you to keep everything under control. Keeping your COOL will keep you from going down the road.

Predetermine and visualize all case scenarios. Coming up with multiple ways to solve the problem will help you visualize the outcome and pick the safest route to take. Examples of worst-case scenarios your Loved One may have:

a. Slid to the floor from the bed (too heavy to lift yourself, call for help)
b. Fell off the toilet and got stuck by the tub (call the Fire Department)
c. Is having chest pains and can't catch their breath (call the Paramedics)
d. Unresponsive and not breathing (call 911 and perform CPR)

These examples are complex but feasible to overcome. Extra steps come in handy for you to be more prepared. If it is unsafe and YOU FEEL it's NOT safe, DON'T DO IT. Call for help should you decide to do something that may require an extra hand. Always let your sidekick know beforehand, not when the sheet hits the fan.

Support Sidekick

Support from your Sidekick gives you extra hands and half the strength on your end. If your Loved One slid off the side of the bed and is now sitting on the floor and there is no physical pain, you can call your sidekick to help you pick them up off the floor.

If, unfortunately, you don't have a sidekick, non-emergency medical help will become your best friend. Try not to call unless needed. Not quite sure whether they bill for excessive service use. Definitely call emergency medical if the injury is worse or there is physical pain.

A.P.E. Method for EMS

Know the proper procedure for calling paramedics and what to do.

Assess your Loved One to ensure you need EMS (Emergency Medical Service) before calling.

Phone 911 and tell them Medical Emergency

Emergency Checklist.

When an emergency occurs and you are waiting for the paramedic, please take these steps.

Emergency Checklist

1. Make sure your Loved One is safe and secure where they are and a pillow is under their head. If you step away, give a blanket if it's cold.

2. Put away any animals in the back room or outside. Keeping them separate will keep both the animals and the medics safe.

3. Retrieve I.D. and Insurance card for Loved One.

4. Have a list of medications with the dose amount available.

5. Clear a path from the door to your Loved One as wide as possible for medic + gurney.

6. Remove any restricted clothing (sweaters) and cover your Loved One with a blanket

7. Be sure the front door is open and the outside light is on if you have one.

8. If you suffer from a language barrier, some translation applications should be available on your cell phone or computer to ensure you are getting the proper care you need.

Measures must be taken, including religiously washing your hands with antibacterial soap before and after any task in conserving you and your Loved One's health.

Is there another enemy besides others who can jeopardize that?

Yes. A mole, YOURSELF. Yup, Yourself!

With you not even knowing it! Sometimes, you will subconsciously set yourself up for failure; the funny thing is, you watched yourself do it. For instance, you open the cabinet and something falls out. You bend down to pick it up and when coming back up, you hit the top of your head on the door you left open. I am not trying to jinx you. Be aware of your safety precautions by "closing that door before bending down."

Ask yourself these questions before and during your resolution of any issue:

1. What is the Issue? (Problem)
2. What do you want? (Result)
3. How to make it happen? (Task)
4. Am I being set up? (Possible task flaws)
5. If so, how to prevent? (Direct task plan)
6. What do you need? (Tools and Supplies)
7. What's the plan, Stan? (Prep materials in order of use)
8. What's next? (Follow your step-by-step order until you have completed your task) Mortal Combat voice-over, "FINISH HIM!"
9. Clean the mess you made

*FRUIT: Step back from the box to think outside of it, it gives you fresher eyes.

Try to think outside the box to be more innovative and see other options you didn't see before.

Chapter 3: LOCC, Meals, Meds and Wound Care

Please understand that anything you need to do for an infant or toddler, you are going to do for your Loved One and more. The only difference is that they can decide for themselves (if possible). Because they're not actual children but REAL adults, like any adult, they deserve to be treated with respect and keep whatever dignity they have left.

*FRUIT: One's level of care will change, but your Loved One's dignity never lessens.

So please tell them about every task you're going to do because people dislike surprises.

They can also help you vs. you struggling to do it all yourself. (Hey, I promote independence and feel people like doing as much as possible for themselves. This way, they won't feel as bad about what they can't.)

Just FYI: You can deal with three types of people; The Compliant, The Compromiser, and/or the Complicator (or Contrary). Depending on who you are dealing with should determine your approach at every task because they can switch on you, depending on their mood.

*FRUIT: The three traits of you: the Compliant, the Compromiser, and the Contrary. Which one will you be today? Keep in mind Murphy's law.

Levels of Care and Consistency (L.O.C.C)

The physical disadvantages are categorized into the three most common stages. Even though there are six primary stages, with more defined care levels, I will focus on the three.

Levels of Care

Levels of Care	Physical Care	Ambulation	Food Consistency	Feed
1	Self Assist	Self Assist	Regular	Self Feed
2	Semi Assist	Semi Assist	Mechanical Soft (Chopped)	Semi Assist
3	Full Assist	Full Assist	Puree (Blended)	Full Assist

Physical care for oneself has three levels; Self, Semi Assist and Full Assist. Care is the normal things like dressing, hygiene, toileting, etc.

Ambulation (or "Mobile") shows levels one through three on whether your Loved One can run amuck alone. You'll need to keep your running shoes on, with a walker or wheelchair nearby.

Don't think that people considered "Bedbound" want to live there, get them out often and it will brighten their spirits a bit.

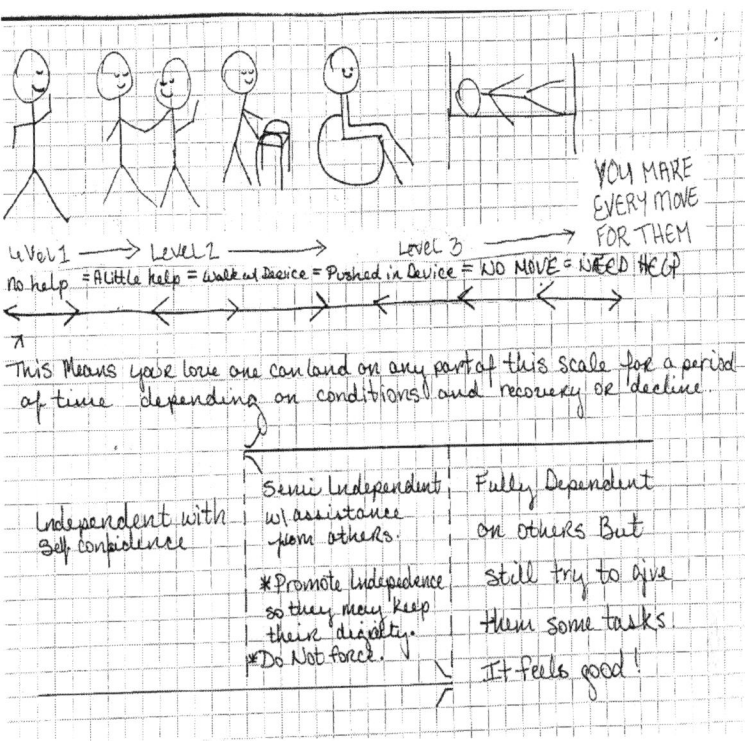

And again, in all the levels of care, you still need to consider their conditions and make changes to accommodate. Many people are bedbound but are able to do for themselves. They just can't walk to the fridge to get their meal. Again, it depends on their condition for the amount of care.

*FRUIT: Nothing is always as it seems. Some people may know how to walk, but not how to eat, speak, or just do…or in any combination thereof. Looks can be deceiving and we remember about ASSUME? Don't assume just because we can do it, your Loved One can as well.

*FRUIT: Please keep in mind, unless these people wear hearing devices, just because they are older or disabled in some way doesn't make them deaf. Stop yelling in their ears! You people know who you are. If that is your normal voice, ok. For others, there's no excuse.

Food Consistency

Along with levels of care, there are also one through three on food consistency.

Food Level One – Regular

- No modifying of food for consumption. This doesn't mean they can tear a steak with their teeth. At least help cut their meat. Well, ask them.

Food Level Two – Mechanical Soft

- Food processed for portioned bites to prevent choking. This is chopped food, so there is some relief in chewing. I chew my food until I know I can swallow. They may chew for a while and it gets tiring. We don't want them to hurry and swallow before it's time and choke.

Food Level Three – Puree

- Food blended to paste consistency for people who choke easily. These people more than likely can't chew at all and just swallow their food once it enters their mouth. Sometimes liquid is also hard to consume since it's so easy for it to go down the wrong tube. I should know.

Not funny, either.

What helps with that is a white powder called Thickener. Add it to any liquid a little at a time to form the right thickness, lowering the choking risk. Now I think they have jelled packets that dissolve better. So, you have your option.

*Keep in mind someone can be ambulatory/mobile but can need puree food. Again, everyone is different.

By YOU knowing what levels of care and food consistencies are, you can now determine where your Loved One stands (or lays) and give them the proper care needed. This also helps you with what adjustments you must make to fit your Loved One's care.

You also need to know if your loved is a Self-Feed or Feed-Assist.

Levels of Self Feed to Feed Assist is the same as Levels of Care

Level One - Self Assist

- Means what it says, they feed themselves. And I hope I feed myself to the very end. Because I love to eat, I think I speak for everyone at some time in their life when I say that.

Level Two - Semi Assist

- Usually means they can assist themselves with supervision. Proceed with caution.

Level Three - Full Assist

- Just what it says as well. When they can't do for themselves. As an example, it's when they need help eating and must have someone to feed them.

They often have a device that may help their independence, such as a modified utensil. Putting a washcloth around the handle and taping it can also be a makeshift/modified utensil.

Meals

(Absolutely NEEDED!) A Course in Heimlich would be suggested and maybe refreshers if you give care for the long term. Go ahead and get the whole thing. It's called First Aid and CPR class.

Mealtimes are crazy, Yo!

Okay, so everyone is picky in their little way and if they could get up to make breakfast, "A" special for themselves, they would. A lot of the time, people complain about the food and become a real princess about it! To avoid all that, you need to sit with them beforehand and ask about all the basic foods they like a particular way.

Snooty Booty *Was only mentioned to avoid any unnecessary arguing. Good Luck with that.

Meal Preparations is learning your Loved One's likes and dislikes and helps give fast and more efficient care. Plus, a chance at a full ten-minute break, you know what I'm saying? I've probably had to remake sandwiches twice before. I learned that fast. Ask what they like and give them what they want. (Needs first)

Keep in mind dislikes and allergies. Mostly just allergies. Some people don't like healthy food, but under these circumstances, I only care that you're not pushing them into anaphylactic shock.

My dad has to ask the restaurant if they fry or cook their fish in the same place as all the other food. Sometimes we won't be able to eat in the first place we stop.

Some foods cause inflammation and other types of flare-ups so be sensitive to what the body reacts to.

On top of this, please cook all food thoroughly and seal it away correctly. We don't poison of any kind, including mold. Be aware of the temperature of the plate and the food.

So, I suggest making the food hot and then letting it sit for five minutes. Precutting the food before serving will give it time to cool down enough and let your Loved One keep what's left of their energy.

Eyeball the leftovers and notate the percentage of the missing pie. If she ate 60% of lunch, make it easy to document, like 60/100.

- Know their allergies
- Portion Control Pie Graph for each individual
- Some need more protein than others

Example
- 50% Veggies
- 25% Protein
- 25% Fruits / Grains

*TIP: Eat when they eat and make sure you prepare an actual meal for yourself. Don't just finish what they left behind. Remember, if you don't care for yourself, there won't be anyone to care for your Loved One. You both will be up the creek without a paddle.

Eating Arrangements

Serving water with every meal and their favorite beverage will help them make the right decision should something go wrong. Sometimes people need help eating, so you might have to feed them. If this happens, wait until they finish chewing, before offering a drink every couple of bites. Please set a certain amount of time aside to help them. Don't rush them because you didn't manage your time correctly. The size of the spoon or fork controls portioned bites. If the whole thing is covered, STOP! That's too much, King Kong. Try to cover only half or less each time.

If they start choking, make it less.

Forget about time altogether.

***FRUIT: Be Patient, my friend, while times occur.**

No shoveling! Give them time to chew. No one wants to rush their meal. You go to a restaurant and eat in your own time. If they rush you, you'll make a scene and won't tip. I'm sorry you will not get tipped in this situation, but you might hear about yourself afterward.

Straws are the shiznit! Go out and stock up. This great creation releases stress on the spilling factor. It also reaches the very last without tipping the cup on someone. They are used for many purposes, but I found them more helpful in limiting the amount given. Simply take the tip of a finger and put it over a straw already in the drink. The suction keeps the fluid in the tube; this way, you can take it out and put it in your Loved One's mouth, giving a good portion of the liquid to swallow.

Now if your Loved One doesn't desire to eat, don't force them. You don't know what's going on in their body. Instead, offer an appetite stimulant, though you may need to Google if you're not familiar with what works.

Depending on the individual and what is best suited for their needs, sit down and have that conversation with your Loved One about the times they would like to eat by or around.

Try to work medications around eating times. If we work it around the meds, it will feel obligated. And people hate the feeling of obligation. Remember to go with the flow if it's hard.

Eating arrangement with mealtimes and meds. Not just:

Breakfast, Lunch and Dinner but also:

- Coffee/Tea
- Brunch
- Supper
- Late Supper
- Night Cap (No Meds)
- Midnight Snack

Slipping meds around then, they hardly put up a fight.

These times are the best time to enjoy each other. Whether it's during a movie or you're the one doing all the talking. We don't want them to choke, okay? Bonding brings you closer and food brings everyone together, so eat together. I hope you enjoy these moments because they will be remembered. Keeping the food near your Loved One's mouth helps with spills and messes. This is common for people needing assistance. Keep a hand towel nearby for unexpected spills or just a bib.

Placing a hand towel over their chest on the runway is a thumbs-up. This is for everyone, including me. They keep dropping food on their lap if the towel is long enough. This is not saving it for later. You can put the other end of the towel under their plate and have a net for the runaway goodies.

They are not suggested for arm flingers.

Repositioning them into an upright sitting position will reduce the chances of choking and make them feel more comfortable eating. This is a given. People don't feel that hungry if they are unable to eat comfortably. So, before all meals, please position them right and ready to eat.

Right and Ready is sitting comfortably with an upright posture and a 90% angle bend at the hips. Use a gait belt, a draw sheet, or just tell them to sit up to help get them in this position. The eating process cohesively works with breathing, lowering the risk of aspiration. (Choking your brains out)

*For people who can't sit still like me sometimes, putting the tv on or background music will distract the little guy inside the brain.

Keep your Loved One's Teeth, Ears, and Eyeballs

The bedside table is used in both the hospital and home setting. So is a tray. Placing things on the tray will help the professionals know what to discard and keep.

Ex. All the things left on top of the tray that was brought in are usually discarded or taken away. So, whatever you plan to keep on the table, take it OFF the tray and put it on the side of the table that is less used. Most commonly, people with dentures lose them this way because they were set down on the tray and then taken away (especially if they're wrapped in a napkin). They'll think, "oh, that's trash." I have heard many stories of people's teeth walking away. Yes, they did.

Remember, what's left on the tray gets thrown away, so watch what goes there.

I have an ironic story to tell you. My mother-in-law thought she lost her partial retainer from leaving it on a tray. We found it twenty years later, in a pants pocket.

Other things to go missing are; glasses, watches, phones, phone chargers and even wallets. So, keep those eyes peeled like a banana.

***TIP:** If your Loved One has to go to the hospital, please leave glasses, hearing aids, dentures, and/or any other prized possessions at home, depending on their length of stay as these things are the most commonly lost or misplaced. If they must go with your Loved One, ensure they're kept in a safe space.

Did you know?

People can burp three ways: normal, through the G-Tube, and through a Colostomy bag (poo bag). Be specific if dealing with these and learn how to deal with them properly. I also heard a hiccup was a lost fart, but it's just a spasm in the diaphragm.

*If the food tray returns with more leftovers than usual, ensure their condition hasn't changed and they can still feed themselves. I saw my father-in-law in a rehabilitation center and noticed he hadn't touched his food. It was then we found out he couldn't use his arms anymore and the facility didn't stay long enough to make sure he was good and able to eat. So please, always wait to leave until after they take a bite of food. Now some people can't have food and we call that:

Nothing Per Oral (NPO), aka nothing by mouth, is for anyone with swallowing issues.

Doctors instruct people of NPO for medical restrictions and pre/post-surgical procedures. It is for the safety of the patients that they follow the NPO guidelines, so no choking occurs (aspiration)

Total Parenteral Nutrition (TPN) is a way to feed people nutrition through the nose who are refusing to eat or are unable to get nutrition through regular diets.

No one should be rushed through eating and drinking. This is where choking is most common, so slow your roll.

Thickener is a drink solution to thicken the drink to the right consistency to avoid aspiration (choking).

G.I. Feeding Tube. I think it stands for Gastral Intravenous. This is an alternative for nutrition intake when all other options are obstructed. Sounds fancy, huh! Feeding times should be scheduled with this because it sometimes will take longer. When this is ordered, I need you to follow the instructions from the physician. Please ask to have a hands-on tutorial. Exact words. Your Loved One's feeding session settings vary from other Loved Ones. Please keep your Loved One in the Fowlers Position which means they are no lower than a 45-degree angle in elevation. Anything lower than that can cause aspiration or choking.

If you can, try and get ahold of an I.V. Pole which holds the feeding bag AKA a kangaroo bag.

Medications

Disclaimer!!!

I told you I am a CNA, NOT a nurse. So, I can't speak about kinds of medicines and or quantity to take. If unsure about medications and need more information, please talk to your nurse or physician. What I CAN speak on is how you take it. Now there are a lot of medicines out there and types.

*Please read the DONT'S before you go and start messing around with your pills.

***FRUIT: If you don't want to read the instructions, fine don't. But you better read the "Do Not." It is necessary and important. A hard head makes a soft bottom.**

DONT'S

*Do NOT, I repeat, DO NOT CRUSH a TIME RELEASED pill. You'll end up giving them the whole thing all at once. JUST DON'T DO IT!

Pills coated in Enteric, when crushed can cause damage to the lining of the stomach. I believe I was told that the coating is to keep it from releasing too early so it can reach beyond the stomach. These also you DO NOT CRUSH.

DON'T give your Loved One anything without first knowing what you are giving. Should there be a time when you don't know if medicine was given and you are thinking about giving them the medication just in case it wasn't? I rather you did not give them the medicine at all versus them dealing with an overdose.

If choking is clear and they need around-the-clock medicine, you might want to inquire about a CADD Pump. It stands for Computerized Ambulatory Delivery Device which is an IV injected automatically and stays connected to the patient. It's a little box with medicine inside and the nurse comes out regularly to change out the medicine cartridge.

Types of Medications

First and foremost, I would invest in a medication minder that is refilled at the beginning or end of every week.

- **Pill** (Compressed Powder)

Ok, compressed powder is usually swallowed whole and sometimes found underneath your Loved One. Slippery suckers slide through fingers and Loved Ones can easily think they took it already, especially if they are taking more than one. You should hang around until after they are done taking them. One pill might try to escape and head down south. (LOL)

If they can't swallow, you can crush them— (Not all). Grind them down to loosen the powder and put them in a small cup, bowl, or ramekin. Powder can be added to a liquid drink, preferably a small glass. They may not be able to drink a whole sixteen-ounce glass, so think about how much they WILL consume. Shot glass will do. What's most popular is applesauce. Anything like applesauce (yogurt and pudding is the shiznit!) Please ensure that when you give it, cover the powder with the food for the bite. Once they taste it before the food, they will be on to you and never trust you with applesauce again.

Oh, it can happen and it has.

- **Pill** (Capsuled Powder)

This goes the same with the compressed. Open it carefully and pour on top.

*derlines**TIP:** When opening the capsule, put a paper of some sort to catch whatever you spill under your medicine.

- **Dissolvable / Chewable**

is self-explanatory. Under the tongue or chew it. Again, if they can't let it dissolve or cannot chew, treat it like a thickener and put it in the shot glass mixed into liquid. It might be different for you.

- **Liquid**

Oral medicine works faster than compressed or capsule because it takes a minute to dissolve into the bloodstream. IVs (intravenously) work even quicker than that because it's directly injected into your bloodstream. However, at home, you don't use IVs. They usually visit the hospital, or an RN will come out. But any who. Liquid is consumed and normally it is given under the tongue or swallowed. Now the stuff is nasty tasting, I know, but there is a trick that I had to use on my mom. Take the syringe and pull a little bit of juice or soda up to a measurable amount. Then pull up the medicine. After that, fill the syringe with more juice or soda. Then say, Mom, want some soda? I'm just kidding. Don't lie to them. Just don't tell them (just kidding).

Alright, alright. Only if they ask.

- **Syringe / Shot**

Most common for diabetics with Type II diabetes.

If your Loved One is unable to swallow and chokes easily, medicine still must be given, so put the syringe (without a needle) on the side of the mouth and massage the cheek around. It helps to enter bloodstream faster.

- **Intravenous** – liquids through a port of some type, whether it be a hep-lock, pick line or the port by the artery in your chest. To the left or right, straight into your bloodstream.

- **CADD Pump** is a machine to give a timed dosage of liquid medication intravenously.

- **G-Tube** – Surgery to bypass your esophagus and straight to the stomach for digestion and nutritional intake. Your stomach breaks the food down and then sends the nutrition through to the other places that need it next for processing. The esophagus is used to break down the intake making it easier for the stomach to digest thus the G-Tube is taking the place of the esophagus.

- **TPN** - Liquid nutrition pumped into your stomach through a line entering your stomach through your nose.

For Your Journal Book Medicine Log

- Date and time
- Issue
- Treat Dosage of what and how much at what time? Was it resolved? And the time it was resolved. If necessary.

Check and recheck the medications when adding more. They might be taking two different medicines for the same thing. All medications need to be re-evaluated for further use or discontinuation in case of conflicting (bad side effects) or duplicating medications. Please consult your physician and/or pharmacist about all medications. If you have a pharmacy error, please take a picture and consult with the professional who handles the medication orders.

Wound Care

Now and then, some people are discharged home and it just so happens they go home with a wound. A wound is an open pressure sore where the skin is broken open to show the other layers of tissue; the deeper the wound, the worse it is. You should find this out before coming home and when you physically assess your Loved One. If this is the case, I suggest you learn about the type of wounds, supplies needed, and care techniques that will help heal the wound and for any future wounds that should arise.

What can take two hours to develop and get worse over a little bit of time will take two months to reduce or even longer to disappear.

Skin Tears

Most common due to thinning of the skin and medications. When blood smuggles its way through the layers of skin, it divides and conquers the area with just the help of a corner wall, for example. You usually just clean the wound and secure it with a covered bandage so the wound doesn't worsen. Do not pull or cut the ripped skin off. Try to put it back over after cleaning it and then bandage it appropriately. If the skin is unable to go back over the wound, or hurts, put a bandage with a generous amount of antibiotic cream and bandage away from the air. This happens mainly on the arms and legs. Bruised skin is the blood pooling between the top layers of skin and, if hit just slightly, can tear like tissue paper and look bad. It just needs to be tended to and protected.

Pressure Sores

The boniest prominent areas on the body are usually where the wounds show up, but there are times when people deal with injuries with cartilage or even in a swollen area. This should be monitored so you can report them to the professional helping with these conditions.

If the professional is aware and schedules wound care, it is usually one to two times a week, but the ones more severe will be dealt with daily.

I have taken care of wounds as small as a scab to the toes falling off. So trust me when I say take care.

The boniest areas consist of, but are not limited to;

- Ears and possibly the back of the head. CRAZY, RIGHT?
- Shoulder blades
- Elbows
- Wrists and hands (don't forget the fingers)
- Hips/Pelvis
- Coccyx / Tailbone (Butt Bone)
- Knees/sides of knees
- Ankles
- Heels
- Sides of feet
- Tip of the toes
- Any area that bends at a joint or has applied pressure constantly. This is a game, find the areas specified?

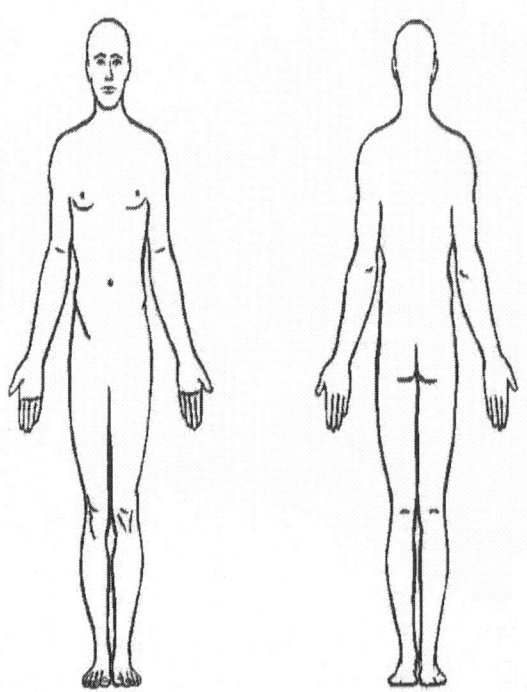

These areas will break down and are measured in stages.

Stage 1

Purple bruise-looking tells you that there has been no blood flow for an extended period and has damage underneath the skin. What usually can occur within two to six hours can take two to six months to heal. There is no accurate healing time because everyone's regeneration is different, so it goes with a range of healing conditions contributing to the slow pace.

Non-blanchable redness. This means when pushing on it, the visible blood flow is not there. Your best bet to deal with this is to take the pressure off of it as much as possible and put protective cream of some sort, then leave alone until it goes away.

Stage 2

The sore is open (broken skin), pink, and has no dead tissue yet, but it is breaking down. Repeat stage one, but you will need to clean it with wound cleanser and dry it with sterile gauze and cover it. Your professional may ask to put medicine on before covering it. Sometimes I think letting it dry out helps; however, do what your professional recommends.

Stage 3

This is where the wound is bigger, having dead tissue and the wound is tunneling underneath, getting deeper. It will show the fatty tissue. Still, keep it clean and cover it. The professional may pack it a little with gauze. This will need changing every time it looks soiled through.

Stage 4

This wound now shows tendon and bone and needs to be packed and covered and may have more of a stench.

Stage 5

There is no stage five. It is just considered unstageable because it has surpassed the stages and needs daily care by a professional. It cannot be categorized because the wound under the surface has tunneled and they can't gauge where or how big unless it opens all the way. Either way, it passes the regular stages. This is hard to keep clean and very painful. It is also one of the reasons people can go septic (infection in the blood) and possibly die.

All these stages are hard to heal, but if caught sooner, you can put you and your Loved One's mind at ease.

I have seen many wounds and at times they have looked like they could cause the demise of a few. If you are dealing with serious wounds, please don't take them lightly.

If they are retaining a lot of fluid in the body and their skin is weeping, leaking clear fluid, this fluid is not pee. This is the body letting go of water because it has nowhere else to go.

FYI- Dealing with fungus and dry skin, or even prolonged wet skin, is the gateway drug for sores to come about.

Chapter 4: Medical Equipment & Devices

With power comes great responsibility. So does taking care of your Loved One. When you move, they move; when you get up, they get up. The same as, when they walk, you walk and when they fall, you fall. Let's understand that when your Loved One does fall, please DON'T stop them. It sounds mean, but it's true. Trying to hold them up puts you at risk and then, in fact, you both fall and are out for the count.

Instead, only catch them to HOLD as you EASE them to the floor. You are protecting them, not from going down, but from slamming to the floor HARD. It saves you a long night in the ER, preventing bone breaks and even sustaining your life. Most of the time, bone breaks are the start of any downfall.

Most important! "Skid socks" or socks with shoes. You must put these items on their feet if they walk, move, or transfer. Depending on the floor you are working with will determine what you use. Sometimes people work better with nothing on, but you figure out what works best for your Loved One and the floor is dry along with their feet. There are other devices out there. However, the list I will speak on is the most popularly used for repositioning, transfers, and ambulation. We call this Durable Medical Equipment (DME) for most that need a physician's order to have covered by insurance. Some, you can get over the counter.

* Please use devices with caution and be aware of the worst possible case scenarios, so you may prevent them from happening. CHECK< CHECK <CHECK!!!!

Dropping someone doesn't feel good and your Loved One? It will kill you inside. Knowing they hurt from your mistake will sit with you. Just keep that in mind. No one is perfect and I should know. You can't be a caregiver for as long as I have and NOT drop anyone or be right there, a second too late, as they fall. Oh boy the guilt, but this is why you learn from my mistakes and never let yourself make that a possibility in the first place.

Emergency equipment helps you know where your Loved One is internally and relay back to the professional helping you.

There are many items that I may not cover, but sometimes, it feels like there is not enough time in the world to cover all of them. When a situation arises, that you don't have what you need, search the problem and find alternative routes and things recommended.

These devices are, but are not limited to:

Vital Equipment

1. **Oximeter**
    a. Little machine that goes on the finger, toe, or ear and reads the oxygen saturation level and heart rate per minute. Most common fits on your finger or toe. It will read the oxygen percentage and pulse. The nickname for this item is "pulse-ox."
2. **Blood Pressure Cuff**
    a. Depending on the type of machine you got, it goes on the wrist, upper arm, or a manual one, with a stethoscope. This tells you the blood pressure (ideal is 120/60) and pulse. Beats per minute (ideal rate is between 60 to 80)

3. **Thermometer**
    a. Tells the temperature. You have the one that slides across the forehead, the one that goes under the tongue, in the armpit, or the rectum. Forehead for me, please. (ideal temp is in the higher 98-degree percentage. Ex. 98.6 or 98.7)
4. **Glucose Meter**
    a. Machine that reads blood sugar levels mostly used by diabetics. This will also help with emergency checks of your Loved One's bizarre behavior and physical actions, or lack thereof. This will assist with your process of elimination to find out what may be wrong, if anything.

Oxygen Equipment

We can't live without oxygen and some of us need help in that department. All devices need to be handled appropriately and watched for problems to come. One being that oxygen can be highly flammable, so be sure to take precautions when using it.

Such devices consist of the list below, but are not limited to:

1. **Concentrator**
    a. Metal tank filled with oxygen, portable for travel.
    b. It only holds so much oxygen that you may need more than one for an outing. No longer than an hour, depending on how many liters you use per bottle.

    c. Machine used to pump room air. Usually pumps up to five to ten liters consistently. If more liters are needed, sometimes, they can connect two, but anything after that, you may need to seek medical attention.

    d. Like all hardworking machines, this machine has a filter on it somewhere. Please pull it off and rinse it under water, ringing it out thoroughly before putting it back.

    e. Please keep this device two to three feet away from the walls and out of any closets. I know it's noisy, but it beats a fire. These things produce a lot of heat and over some time will heat the surroundings.

    f. Portable Concentrator- Same as above, just compact. (Carry or get a second battery. I can't recommend it enough.)

*TIP: With the heat escaping, a concentrator keeps a room warm for the "cold-blooded."

2. Tank

    a. Portable oxygen tank for outings that can come in sizes big, medium, and small. Like Goldilocks, find what's just right.

3. Regulator

    a. Device connecting the tank to the cannula. This regulates how much oxygen is released. One is continuous release and the other only releases when a breath is taken. This one prolongs the use and wastes less oxygen. It comes with a key that looks like a fake bottle opener.

b. Please ask the professionals to give you a quick tutorial on how to change tanks. Remember "righty tighty, lefty loosie". Don't get this confused with Tidy Whities.

4. **Canula**
    a. Tubing connecting to an oxygen machine of some type.
    b. This tubing has two ends like a fork facing into the nose and then loops around the ears in front. I understand it can be annoying, so loosen it. I never recommend having it go around face from behind. This is only in the movies for looks. This will turn into a noose and can possibly restrict your Loved Ones breathing if are unaware. This is what the oxygen flows through to get to your Loved One. The two-holed prongs release the air directed straight up the nose.
    c. Do not put it around the head to keep it on. It can slide down and become a noose very quickly. Not cool. Instead, put prongs into nostrils and then guide the hose up and around both ears following it down to the throat. Reaching where the hoses meet is a tightener. Push it up to the throat loosely.
    d. The canula is usually seven feet long and connects directly to the concentrator or regulator for a tank. Other feet lengths include twenty-five feet and fifty feet. Anything longer that is needed ask for a

"Christmas tree" extender piece that will connect two hoses making it one longer one.

e. There are face masks available but a lot of the time, our Loved Ones feel claustrophobic with it on.

f. If they are mouth breathers, put the canula with the prongs facing in the mouth, so they can still get the oxygen while they sleep.

5. **Oxygen Mask**

   a. Mask connects to cannula.

6. **Rebreather mask**

   a. Mask with a bag connected to reserve oxygen for a bigger breath.

7. **Humidifier**

   a. To be clear I am talking about the extra device that comes with the concentrator. This hooks from the machine to the canula and then the canula to your Loved One. It should be filled 1/3 high with distilled water. Now please don't forget to refill it when low. If filled too high, the water will make it up the nose of your Loved One and into their lungs. The air will still be dry through the humidifier with no water. Just remember, one more water dish to fill or plant to water. Make it a routine to check levels and refill. This is something that helps with the dry air forced through the nose. That is why people are eager to use Vaseline in the nose. Well, please don't. Look for something petroleum free.

b. It is a device connected to a sterile water tube and helps the oxygen pass through to keep the air hydrated enough so the nose doesn't dry out. Reduces the possibility of nose bleeds.

c. Keep all flammable things away and post a sign about oxygen in use if needed.

8. **Nebulizer**

a. Machine turning liquid medicine to vapors for breathing treatments such as steroids.

Hospital Bed & Bedside Table

1. **Manual** (Crank) Bed (The back breaker)

a. A manual crank at the end of the bed (Watch your shins!) that raises the bed in height, head and feet. These are about to become obsolete, but I tell you what. In a power outage? I would be thanking my stars for this classic beauty.

2. **Electric**

a. Remote-controlled bed. It deals with height, head and feet. Pay attention to where you leave the remote for this one. Sometimes my grandfather sandwiched himself in the middle of the night. It should be able to hang on the railing or you can rig it.

b. Both should come with a remote control, side rails and locks on the bottom of the feet. If any of these things are damaged, malfunctioning, or missing? Please report it and have it repaired or replaced.

> I. Remote
> II. Rails
> III. Wheel locks

3. Bedside Table
> a. Adjustable height and on rollers so it can slide under the bed to reach in front of your Loved One. The height adjusting leaver is on the side of the post under the table top
>> I. A real mess if it gets knocked over.

Toileting Equipment

These devices are used for toileting and other purposes. Here are the description of the most common:

1. Urinal
> a. Plastic liquid measuring pitcher. You can really use anything for peeing that has handles. Please rinse this out after every use and clean it appropriately. Using vinegar to do the last rinse will keep the smell down.

2. Bed Pan
> a. Standard looks like the top of a toilet seat to poop on in the bed.
> b. Fracture pans are usually for people with hip fractures, breaks or that can't turn over easily. It can also cause more damage. Pay attention to where you place it, not just shove it under them. Skin tears can happen.

3. **Bedside Commode**
    a. Crossbreed between a toilet and a walker. Portable toilet seat with handles and a removable collection bucket. This can be used at the end of the bed, over the toilet seat, and in the shower (preferably without the bucket). These should come with an aim assistant. Wide round tub with no bottom that sits in the same place as the bucket. It keeps everything controlled to go straight in the toilet.

4. **Toilet Seat Riser**
    a. Seat riser that sits in place of the toilet seat. While some come with handles, consider the ones to match your Loved One. Some are less stable than others.

5. **Catheter** - It is imperative to keep the catheters clean and flushed by a professional when needed. I think once a week is normal, but please look into this. The bag itself can be changed once every week or two. If you smell it, change it.
    a. **Standard** - (Foley) Device opens the pathway for urine internally. It's a balloon that seals the canal and contains while drains. The tube will protrude from the tip of a man's penis or out the urethra of a woman.
    b. **Condom** - The one that's external use only. It's a condom with adhesive and a hole in it. I speak for all the men when I say this one can hurt when it's being changed because it may pull pubic hair.
    c. **Pubic** - Tube surgically protruding from the pubic area.
    d. **Rectal** – this device is to catch the BM that continuously comes out because of incontinence. Also

used to collect stool samples for testing. This is rare to receive.

6. **Colostomy**
   a. Surgical incision to bypass an area in the digestion track. The poo will come out this way in the meantime. It is covered with an adhesive collection bag that is emptied or replaced when soiled or full. Sores and redness can occur with this if not cleaned properly. The bacteria in poo eat our skin.

*TIP: These things need to be burped. I know, crazy analogy, right? Burped like a baby, releasing the air from the bag. If you don't, they will pop like the stink bomb my brother put in the Christmas tree during the opening of presents.

Output/Specimen Catcher

1. **Foley bag**
   a. Collection bag connected to the end of the catheter.
   b. To empty this, you need a graduate or a container. Usually, you can tell the valve is open when the right side is sticking out more. But all manufacturers make them slightly different. Examine the one you got.
   c. Please don't forget to close it.
   d. Put something down to protect your floor underneath.

2. **Leg bag**
   a. Is the same as a Foley bag, but straps to the leg.
   b. Usually has a twist cap valve.
   c. Please remember to close the valve after every use.

d. Ensure the bag is empty before dressing. Put the bag through the pant leg before their actual leg.

3. **Graduate**
   a. Is another type of urinal. However, you will use this for the emptying of the pee bag. You can also use any other type of container to empty if you are not having to measure the output of pee. You can also use the regular urinal if need be.

4. **Hat**
   a. Elimination collector and measurer. This is commonly for people under output observation. Comes in really handy though. If barely used, bleach well and save it for more specimen needs in the future. It looks like a hat and goes upside down on the toilet rim and under the seat.

5. **Specimen cup**
   a. Clear cup with screw top for stool or urine sample

Bathing Equipment

I absolutely recommend all of these to be in your home. Of course, I recommend all of it, in this book, but these are used religiously or more often than others. I walked into the house that had nothing and we had to 'MacGyver' it a couple of times. If you have any of those problems and are without, look for alternatives that do the same thing. You don't realize how much you will surprise yourself.

1. **Wash Basin**
    a. Bucket that holds water. Use it for baths and messes. Clean out after every use. It is one of the most common places to hold bacteria and recontamination. If it becomes too dingy, replace it.
2. **Shower Chair** – please research for the right one
    a. Standard Shower Chair
        i. Chair made to sit in the shower and able to get wet with holes in the seat so the water flows.
    b. Sliding Shower Chair
        i. The seat slides in and out of the shower
    c. Chair Bench
        i. Chair Benches are for the more dependent and/or heavy. They spill over the tub wall so you can sit and scoot.
3. **Shower Head**
    a. Getting a special shower head with an extending hose. Blesses shower times to be more pleasant.
4. **Adjustable Handlebars**
    a. Suction handlebars are highly recommended for stability and independence. Please take them off and clean both the suctions and wall. This should be done periodically to rejuvenate the suction. You can also install permanent ones; however, I suggest that they are long and can be reached at any position.

For Oral Care

1. **Dent-Tip Swabs** - This is a stick with a sponge cube on one end. Used to moisturize and clean the mouth, as well as brush teeth. I love these things so please be sure to ask for some.

2. **Emesis Basin** – a new age spittoon shaped like a kidney bean and normally made out of plastic.

Repositioning Equipment

We don't want any breaks and in order to keep that enforced, you need to know the basic safety devices, that will help with repositioning, transfers and or ambulation.

1. **Draw Sheet**
    a. A regular flat sheet - These normally come in your bed sheet set. Depending on what fits you best will be folded different ways for repositioning or transferring. I noticed that I could fold the sheet three ways for beneficial use.
        i. Hamburger - Top and bottom of the sheet is folded together, leaving a smaller yet fatter sheet (also called doubled when used as a top sheet.
        ii. Hotdog - Folding both sides together will make a long skinny draw sheet. This gives you more pulls when scooting your Loved One up in the bed. Granted, this isn't for any of our heavy, Loved Ones. It would be hard to reach around them to grab the sheet if you can barely see it on

the sides. I suggest Hamburger for our heavier Loved Ones.

iii. Standard - Folding the top to the bottom and then from one side to the other giving you four layers, making it more durable in repositioning.

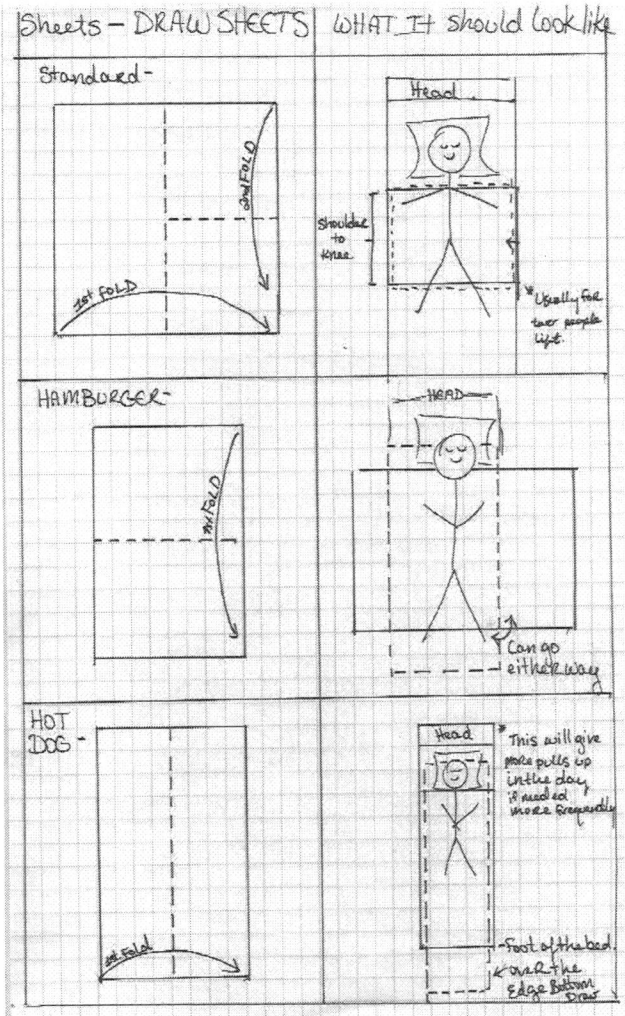

b. These draw sheets come in handy in chairs so that if your Loved One is a recliner sleeping, with this underneath them, you won't have to worry about something happening to them, slipping down and not being able to get them out of the chair. This should be considered a part of your Loved One's body when you have full assistance.

*TIP: Keeping the four ends facing downwards towards the feet, will also keep the wrinkles down behind them.

2. **Cushions** – Any shape and size pillows that help reposition your Loved One. Ones they like. The more, the better.

    a. There are other pillows or cushions made for position required. But I think with a little readjusting and manipulation to the pillow, will get the job done.

3. **Trapeze**

    a. You will not go to the Olympics using this. This is for you Loved One to reposition themselves up higher in the bed or lift up for you to smooth wrinkles out from behind them.

Transfer Equipment

1. **Draw Sheet**

    a. This sheet is only really used for transferring Loved Ones entirely reliant on you. The sheet is to help you pull or lift them. It can be used side by side with the slide board.

2. **Slide Board**

    a. Smooth board (not just any board, don't get crafty with these) helps slide your Loved One into the chair or bed. With the help of the draw sheet, you will have a smoother transfer.

3. **Gait Belt**

    a. Belt goes around your Loved One above waist level and is tight enough to put two fingers through both sides of their body. If you make it too tight, you might get slapped. For the women, please make sure it is under her breast. If men have man boobs, do the same, he might slap you too.

4. **Hoyer Lift**

    a. Electric or manual (hammock-like) machinery that lifts your Loved One out of or onto the chair or bed. The Hoyer part detaches from the hammock and when in a chair, the hammock stays underneath your Loved One's booty. Warning*! Do not use it by yourself. You need two people to operate safely. Now please keep in mind that it is NOT an ambulation device. Don't wheel them around in the Hoyer because the hammock is swinging and the base does not open wide enough to prevent tipping. You can come from many positions; however, the side is safer than the front and if you are a professional, you can use the position from the back. But that is iffy.

    b. The hammock has handles to help hold it and can come with or without a hole in the butt for restroom use. Oh yeah, it looks like a cherry-picker for engines.

Ambulation Equipment

1. **Hemi**
    a. A crossbreed between a cane and a walker. It looks like a walker and yet, you use it like a cane. It's crazy, right?! Use a gait belt in combination for more security.
2. **Walker**
    a. I think everyone knows what a walker is. Also using a gait belt with this will help prevent accidental falls for unstable people.
        i. **Standard -** It's a good idea to get slides that attach to the feet so they glide.
        ii. **All-wheel** with or without a seat and or storage
            1. The breaks sometimes go out so they are only reliant as long as the breaks are working. If the breaks go out, get a new one or get it fixed.
3. **Merry-Go-Round**
    a. Looks like a walker for a child made of PVC piping and a seat for an adult. No room for toys, but may have a tray to help hold items on top. These are not too common. Used mainly for those who are a complete fall risk and needs to be monitored 24/7 and that you're unable to keep a constant eye on.
4. **Wheelchair**

All wheelchairs should come with working breaks, handles to push, armrests for your Loved One and footrests (attached or detachable). They all should be foldable for storing away or to fit in the trunk of your car. If your wheelchair does not come with any of these or is missing a piece, return it to the sender and ask for a complete one.

    a. **Transport**
        i. Chair with wheels small enough to push through narrow doorways. Keep this in mind if I just described your house. The foot pedals may or may not be able to take off.

    b. **Standard**
        i. Chair with wheels big enough for Loved Ones to wheel themselves. Comes with detachable footrests.

    c. **Electric**
        i. A chair with wheels and a motor they can drive in the sitting position.

    d. **Scooter**
        i. Manual push is normally used for people with foot issues.
        ii. This usually has 3 wheels.

    e. **Electric Scooter**
        i. Goes fast. Be careful.
        ii. This is usually a chair with a motor and steering wheel.
        iii. Can come with 3 (possible tipping hazard) or 4 wheels.

Mantra REPO-TRAN-AMBU-ROM-N-OT

My Ode to dance (5,6,7 and 8)

Consider the following chapters a dance routine between you and your Loved One. A beautiful show of fluidity of movement, gliding, magnificent turns, and extensions of the arms and legs to the fingers and toes. These are the five actions you do with your body.

5. Repositioning
6. Transfers
7. Ambulation
8. Range of Motion and Occupational Therapy

All these important sections are to complete: a turn, move, go and keep moving. In these chapters, you will learn how to scooch and roll your Loved One into the position they need while making them comfortable, move them to a specific location, and take them anywhere they want to go. The body in motion will stay in motion. If you stop, contracting of the limbs will debilitate and be painful for you both. Sometimes, this is inevitable, depending on the condition, but trying doesn't hurt.

Some people may feel they don't need such childish help. While they are doing childish things, it does not mean they are a child. Speak to them like the adult they are and let them know it is only a precaution. Blame it on me if you want.

Perform that dance across the clouds.

Chapter 5: Repositioning

What is repositioning?

It means to move into a different position than before, to keep blood flow, prevent long-term wounds, and atrophy of the body.

When we sleep, we normally want to lay down and when we eat, we want to sit up. While we sleep, we don't move unless our body tells us we lack blood flow and a sense of pain to specific areas. With your Loved One, this may not be the case and therefore, needs assistance in moving those parts of the body.

For example:

When your foot is on the bed and the pressure of weight pushes on your heel, blood flow is pushed away from the condensed area. Pinched nerves send signals to the brain, making it register as uncomfortable and then you REPOSITION to a new position that is NOT lacking flow. Until that flow slows down too, then you move again. You're asleep, you don't know. For someone who can't move, the pain stays until it goes numb, but if touched or moved after, extreme pain and then good pain. Good pain means it feels good to move but very painful. We want to try to avoid that.

Although we're asleep, our blood flow slows down along with our pulse. I don't suggest moving them every one to two hours, unless they are on prominent bones and awake. If you want them to sleep well, only move them once or twice and see the pillow positioning section. Now I play the record. If you are constantly vigil, you can let them sleep, but if you lack the continuous check, follow a clock guideline.

Ex.: 8 pm- lay down, Midnight- move position, 4 am- move different position, 8 am- get up. Yes, I know this means you don't sleep well, but you can take turns if you have your Sidekick. The more pillows, the more comfort, less movement, and more sleep for you both.

Position's people lay in are called:

1. Supine – Laying on your back, belly to the sky.
2. Prone – Laying on your face, farts ready to fly.
3. Side - Left or Right Lateral. Just means they are lying either on their left or right side. BOOM!
4. Fowlers - forty-five-degree angle elevated. This is most typical for people with breathing and or digestion issues, such as congestive heart failure or a G-tube/Feeding tube etc.

Elevating the legs before putting them in position 4 will help keep them from sliding down less. Just make sure they are all the way up in bed first. To do that:

Scooting Higher Up in the Bed

Positioning higher in the bed is the most common reposition made ALL day. If the sheet is folded hot dog length (please see the hamburger/hot dog diagram in Chapter 4), the sheet will stay under them longer allowing for more pulls up, towards the top of the bed before you have to reposition the sheet underneath them.

In doing this, you keep them bending at the hip, not the lungs. For heavier Loved Ones, a hamburger style draw sheet will be best so that if you can't do it alone, you and your Sidekick can hold both sides of the sheet.

If they are in a regular bed, you and your Sidekick need to hold the high sides of the draw sheet, count to three, and pull them up in a higher position. With a free hand, still having the drawsheet up where their head isn't touching the bed, position pillows behind them supporting the whole back. This may take more pillows than usual, so keep more nearby.

Put a Chuck (because when it's used, you chuck it) or plastic disposable pad plastic side up underneath the draw sheet. It will help the drawing sheet slide better.

Alternatively, if you don't have a Chuck, open a garbage bag completely to make a rectangle and safety pin the corners to the bed which will make for an easier slide.

This will also mean you must keep their legs elevated slightly so they won't slide down easily.

For a Single Person

This method will help keep them from sliding down in a hospital bed.

When lying flat on their back (supine), pull the pillows out from behind them. If they need to be pulled up because they are too far down, you can do it yourself.

1. Put the head down and the feet up.
2. Repositioning their pillow between the headboard and the top of their head. So, you don't knock them silly.
3. Standing at the head of the bed, reach over your Loved One and grab the sides of the drawsheet close to their body, pushing your stomach against the headboard. Pull your arms back into your body, dragging them

towards you, higher up in the bed. Gravity is our friend and comes in handy sometimes.

    4.   While keeping their feet up, sit them up while slowly lowering their feet.

Don't worry about being strong enough because this is 90% mental and 10% physical when you move smart and use gravity as your friend…ok, maybe 20% physical, but the idea is that it is less strenuous than what you might think.

Scooting Higher in the Chair

In a chair, there should always be a precaution such as a drawsheet underneath them for you or a gait belt secured around them. Then, you may have the help of the drawsheet to scooch your Loved One. In the chair, you may be limited, but moving them can still be done. At least you can still pick them up with the help of the gait belt.

Wheelchair

    1.   Make sure locks are in place before moving them.
    2.   Reaching underneath their arms from behind and grabbing, not their wrists but, the forearms and pull their arms close to their body then up while they push from the floor or foot pedals.
    3.   Your upper chest should be pressed against their back.
    4.   If their arms are limp and you have back problems, or it is just a no-go, put a gait belt on them and, standing in front of them with your knees touching theirs, pull them up while pushing the knees back with yours.
    5.   You can also do #1 with their pants, but this is where wedgies come into play.

6. Using the draw sheet in the chair and having two people (you and your Sidekick), pull each side up on the count of three and towards the back. Ensure your grip is good and close to your Loved One's body.

7. For the strong ones standing from behind the wheelchair, lean on the handles and lift the front wheels as far back as you can, jiggling the chair until their butt slides back farther in the chair. This may be a little jolt for your Loved One, but if they know you will not drop them, they'll get used to your ways. This is for the experienced and strong, who will not drop them. I don't recommend anyone do this if they aren't confident and capable. Don't test unless you know you won't drop them.

In the Bed

Sometimes you can just check on them to see if they are repositioning themselves, but if they are not, move them to the other side softly and let them know you are there. If you're checking them at night, use a night light only as they may get scared and punch what they think is an intruder. No prowlers allowed.

1. Rolling

    a. This is where a draw sheet becomes your best friend. Rolling from one side to the other is sometimes hard, but if you cannot roll them on your own, the sheet will help you with that. This will also ensure you don't injure your Loved One by accidentally grabbing their skin or a wounded area.

    b. While rolling your Loved One, use the sheet to push them to the other side, and if they're able to, ask them to hold the other side to keep themselves rolled over. Keep one hand on the lower back (NOT the HIP). Guide the leg to the opposite side, bracing the back.

  c. Using a pillow between their legs can also help keep their spine and pelvis aligned. The pillow technique is helpful for dealing with breaks, fractures, or pain relief.

2. Positions and Pillows

  a. Keeping the hip aligned by putting a pillow between the knees and ankles. Diagonally - top of thigh to ankle

  b. A pillow in front of them to hold and a pillow in the back to lean on. Very comfortable.

  c. Make sure they are not lying on their arm; the shoulder is out from under them and the pillow bracing head to the shoulder.

Sometimes, too many pillows on the bed can be bad. Some feel suffocated by too many. Only keep what they want or need, up to sixish. One or two for the head, one for the back to lean on, one between the knees to help keep the pelvis aligned, one in the front, and maybe two extras where they feel boney spots.

Pillow(s)

Main thing to know with pillows is:

*Pull the "maid card" and fluff and flip their pillows every three or four hours. They tend to flatten out and can cause more harm than help.

*Some people love sleeping on a bed of pillows. If you close your eyes, it's like clouds.

*Experiment with positions of the pillows, double checking all their possible boney spots protected.

***TIP:** Please, be mindful of their back, shoulder blades, and hips. This is usually where more pressure on the body occurs. Reminder, again, that it's very important to rotate them from supine to left, right, or prone. Not a lot of people are able to be in the prone position for many reasons.

Not many pillows are needed depending on boney areas and comfort, but elevating the legs is most important. There are special cushions that have a hole in the middle called a donut. Even rolling a large towel and shaping it into a donut will suffice as well. In some instances, the towel may even be better than the donut because you can manipulate it to fit your Loved One's behind and comfort. I, myself, sleep with a baby feeding pillow.

Positions with Pillows

There are many pros to using these positions. The cons can be slightly higher with flexibility restrictions and movement sensitivity. Don't force your Loved One into a position that is uncomfortable for them. So, keep pillows near for comfort catchers. There are many ways to place pillows. The positions I will demonstrate are the most common; however, you can manipulate the pillows to their liking and put them anywhere depending on the number of pillows.

Placing pillows in these areas are great.

Back

- Left side
- Right side
- Middle low
- Middle high
- Middle center

Joints

- Between the legs at the knees (this is a side position)
- Under the elbows (boney and needs to be repositioned)
- Under the knees (while laying on your back)
- Under the ankles, floating the heels (also laying on your back)
- Behind the hips. With using two pillows, it helps make a little crevasse where your tailbone is floating in a little bit of air, relieving pressure and allowing blood flow to re-enter the earth's atmosphere of your butt.

SUPINE

Placing a pillow on both sides of the back where the diamond positioned pillows' one corner touches high in the center or low in the center of the back. This leaves a space between the shoulder blades, but still remains cushioned.

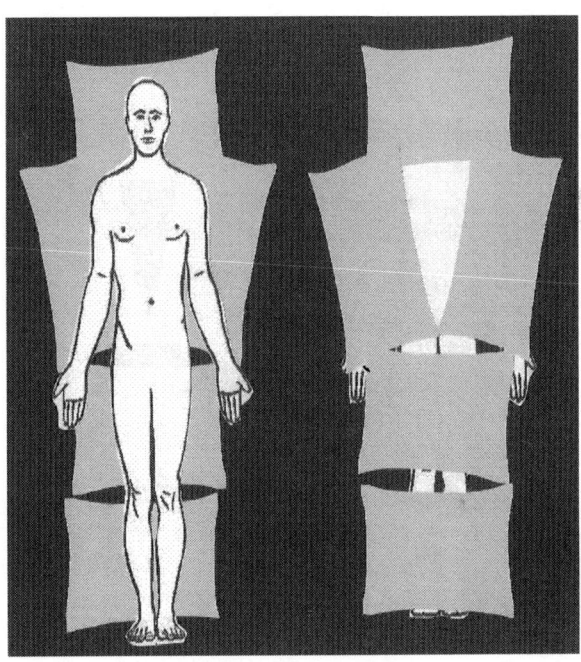

Leaving a little gap in between the pillows, near the tailbone will cradle the bone there and give room for circulation.

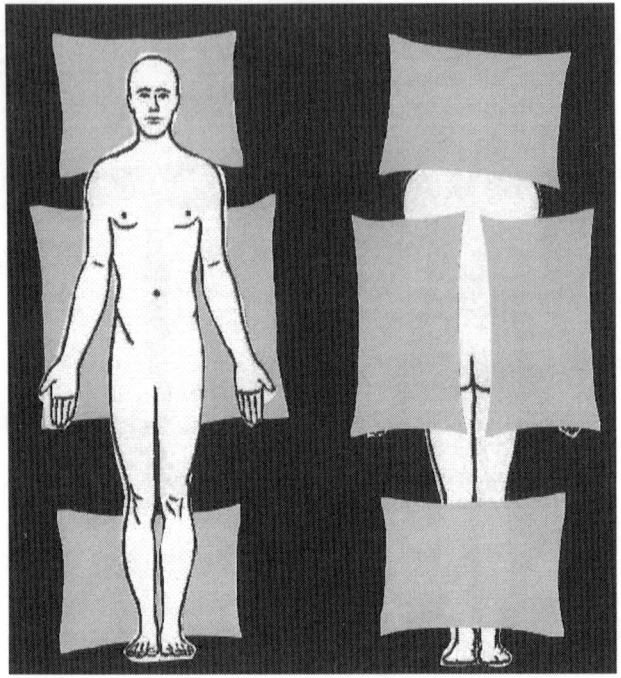

These are just a few of the many ways to position pillows for your Loved One.

PRONE

Pictures were not made in the prone position with pillows because it's very rare for a person to lay on their stomach for extended periods of time.

BI-LATURAL (SIDE to SIDE)

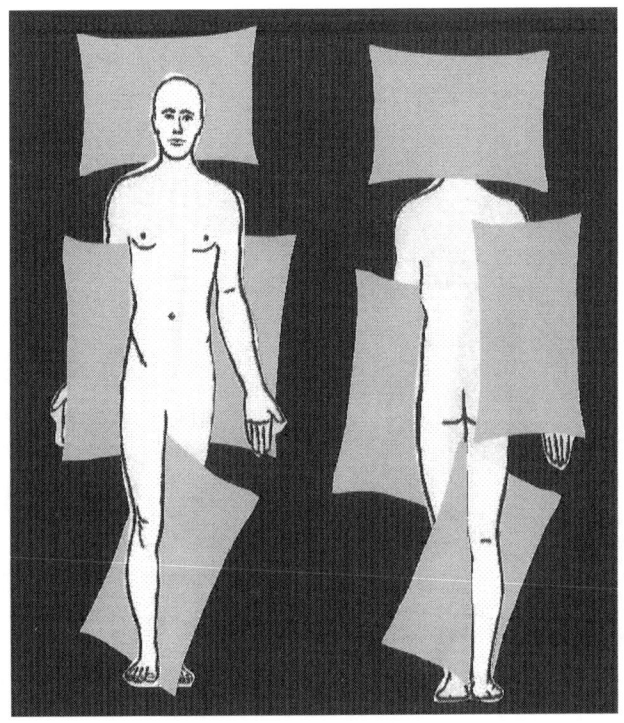

Safety Measure Need to Know

You are on a need-to-know basis and you NEED to know this. It doesn't matter what level of care your Loved One needs. All of them are subjected to falling out of bed. Please take your precautions and consider what you can to keep them safe. If you have a regular bed like most, I suggest getting some type of railing that slides in between the mattress and box spring, so they may hold it while they do whatever they do. If this is not enough, consider some type of nonskid mat you pull out while they sleep. Let them be aware of it before they sleep. Come a time, they wake up and feel something under their feet and try to jump out of the bed. If this happens, they'll land on the mat making for a softer fall.

Using pillows as a barrier is ok but ensure your Loved One is comfortable and doesn't feel claustrophobic.

Precautionary and Safety Placement

Just because you have a bunch of pillows doesn't mean you will always use them for comfort. Placing some pillows under the bed sheets will help reduce the risk of falls or, for runners, give you a head start in hearing them struggle before they make it past that hump in the sheet and out the bed.

Pillows are comfortable meant for the boney parts of your body that hurt or become bruised from flat and firm surfaces.

Using makeshift pillows

If pillows are something that you are lacking at the moment, experiment with rolled towels or blankets as an alternative. Granted, these are denser than pillows, but finding the right one rolled the right way that fits them comfortably, can substitute very well.

Contracted limbs

Rolled towels work for the gap in-between contracted limbs (any limb stuck in a particular position mostly close to the body).

Don't make them too thick, or it will hurt. Also, a rolled washcloth will be suitable for the contracted hands. Nails are often too hard to cut and, therefore, can dig into the skin of their palms.

***TIP:** Please do NOT leave your Loved One sitting unattended at the edge. Make sure if left alone, they are secured in their surroundings.

Follow your environmental precautions and ensure a direct line for help is within reach of your Loved One should you be away longer than expected. If you're leaving home, even for five minutes, something can happen to you, like going unresponsive, and no one would know your Loved One is home alone. Bad news for everybody.

SAVE A MEMBER CHECKLIST

When positioning someone, you can't leave them until you know all limbs are out from under any body weight or tied up in the sheets. And yes, that also includes genitalia. Wedgies are very uncomfortable, you know. For men it may be the scrotum and for women the lower vaginal skin that gets stretched uncomfortably.

Think about; body size, stature, pain levels and pain locations on the body to save the member.

Member List

1. *Arms (keep joints straight and elbows protected with a pillow if possible)*

2. *Hands (open and accessible so they may do what they please with no restraints)*

3. *Fingers and thumbs (not twisted or digging into each other or other parts of the skin)*

4. *Legs (straight and not pushing hip out of place)*

5. *Feet (make sure feet and ankles are not twisted in the sheets)*

6. *Heels (raise the heels and float them by placing a pillow under the ankle, NOT under the heel)*

7. *Toes (weight from the blanket can cause sores on the tips of the toes so prop the blanket up like a tent.)*

8. *Breasts (they can sometimes be stuck under the armpits so be sure to lift them out)*

9. *Testicles (they can get stuck underneath and can hurt so be sure they are in a safe position)*

10. *Underwear (can give wedgies so pull the underwear loose enough but still secured)*

Level of Care

Level one

Less of a responsibility for you since they are more mobile than most, but don't be fooled. If they suffer from forgetfulness, setting timers to reposition or move around is a Godsend.

Maybe it's time for a walk. Ask if they need to use the restroom). Your guidance to the bathroom or where they go should be good ONLY if they are stable. Now I know some days are more unstable than others, so having a gait belt handy is vital; it will accessorize your Loved One's outfit perfectly.

*TIP: Before doing ANYTHING with your Loved One, please keep in the forefront of your mind any object that may be attached to their body, such as a Foley bag, IV, etc. Foley bags tend to hang off something. Just make sure you detach it and keep it near your Loved One. I hang it on the back of the belt so it won't be forgotten.

What are the advantages for these Loved Ones?

Independence fills their pride of still being here. They are not a burden to their family and their dignity never dies. The burden is a hard pill to swallow for them; reassuring them that they're not is so hard to conquer. Asking them if they want to do things with you will let them know that you enjoy their company and feel less of an obligation to you in their eyes.

In the Chair

Leaning on the pillows helps relieve pressure off the bum some and elevating the feet assists blood flow back to the heart. Sitting on a pillow on harder surfaces helps prevent the tailbone from being bruised. As the pillows become smushed, they become a hindrance, so I suggest taking them out occasionally, fluffing them up and reinserting in a few hours.

Level Two

These Loved One's need help but should try to do what they can. You just give them that little extra oomph! Whether it's helping them roll to the side or giving a tug of the hand to sit up, please be gentle. Sometimes people ache and it's not enough for them to tell until you touch it. Make sure it's a gentle one.

Now, this level is like a mix of one and three. Have them roll onto their sides. Get off that booty. A pillow between the legs positioned to fit under the knees and the ankles. A pillow between the knees helps keep the hip aligned. Repositioning is vital when they're not in motion. I figure what takes two to six hours to make takes two to six months to go away. Yes, I'm talking about bedsores. That's why you protect the ankles. If their ankles touch for long periods of time, the boney spots become sore and discolored. This sore eventually opens up, becoming a wound. Or the skin turns black and dies.

So, bathroom visits and transfers can be considered as a turn in your turning schedule.

If sliding is their thing, ensuring they are fully on the bed or chair is a good idea. To make that happen, use a gait belt. Remember to put hands at ten and two (driving wheel) underneath your Loved One's arms and make sure your arms are flexed and strong (no spaghetti arms). This makes your Loved One feel supported and gives them the confidence to know that if they fall, you have them. Knock your knees to theirs and stand shoulder-length apart. Ideally, one knee helps the most. The other is the strength trunk. Now, sit them back. They should be all the way on the seat or bed.

Shoes or socks with grips work as stoppers or prolongers.

To roll over, you should guide the leg, by the back of the knee, to the opposite side in the direction desired.

Wheels should be locked on the bed. If you notice movement, put a rug under them (if none) and then try to be on the side desiring to face and guide them towards you. Then, the bed won't roll away.

*TIP: If you have one side of the bed by the wall and the bed has a railing, put a spacer between the legs of the bed and the wall. This keeps your Loved One from smashing their fingers.

Level Three

"But, what if they want to sit on the edge of the bed?" Well, my dear friend, this is not as complicated as you think.

1. Have your Loved One bend their knees and hold their legs with one arm. Your arm will be positioned over their legs.

2. Scoop under their back and armpits with your other arm. This arm will be positioned under them.

3. Roll them like an egg, first towards you with their feet off the bed.

4. Sit them upright with their feet on the floor. This will keep the spine straight and hips even.

In relation to the egg, your Loved One will roll in the bed during the sitting up process. If your Loved One is a little heavier it will be more complicated. This will be more of a square situation than an egg. So, this is modified to protect you at the same time and back problems sometimes feel they are here to stay, so let's minimize or even prevent them.

1. Roll them facing the edge they'll be sitting on and move their feet off the bed.

2. Then try to reach under their arm and hold their back, helping them sit up.

3. Warning, when people lie down for an extended period of time, their equilibrium will be off and they need a minute to sit up. Dizziness can make them sick, so keep the waste bin near if something surprises you.

Chapter 6: Transfer

Considering you have repositioned your Loved One into the sitting position, I suspect they may feel dizzy from lying down to suddenly up! This is okay. You need to give them a few moments to get acclimated to the new position before you are ready to transfer them. Let them stabilize while you plan the next move.

To move your Loved One from the bed to a chair or other places, I recommend you use one to two of any transfer devices (a gait belt being one), especially on outings to ensure you and your Loved One comes back home and not to the hospital. 100% = 10% Loved One and 90% All, YOU, baby!

You can only fully complete a safe transfer if they have their 10%. Their percentage is a willingness to go through what it takes. This is where your Sidekick can come and help if your Loved One doesn't have 10%.

Keep in mind the **BRACE POINTS** you need. Everywhere your Loved One will reach for, should they become unstable, these brace points should have some type of handle for them to grab. There are many ways to transfer. Using fewer moves would be in the best interest for a safe transfer. To find those brace points is to see any areas your Loved One might fall. This is what your environment setup is primarily for. Your Loved One will grab at all eight angles from them and anything nearby, stable or not. Make sure what they reach for is intended to be there for the safe brace points.

Sit where they sit and pretend you are them. Now, reach out for places you are scared of falling and place a brace point there. Imagine the fall and what would have prevented it if something stable had been there.

Level One

Help them transfer as normal. Should you notice it is an "off" day for them, keep the gait belt around their waist. Remember, no spaghetti arms. A REALLY "off" day, have your Loved One stay still more frequently. Ambulating at these times can result in injury or a doctor's visit. Let's just consider them a level two that day. If you don't have a gait belt, a regular belt will work but hold it near the buckle doubling on the strap with the grasp.

*TIP: If this funk lasts for more than three days, you might need to consider this the new normal if everything else comes out fine. They may snap out of it. Hope for the good, you know. If they don't, make that doctor's appointment.

But if they do it for themselves? Let's make it easier for them and the coach. Direction to move in? Strong side.

Transfer out of bed or chair

1. Make sure the bed/chair is locked and secured.
2. Have them scoot to the edge and feet flat on the floor and shoulder length apart.
3. Lean forward and push up from the bed with a fist or hold onto the chair's armrests until standing straight up. Put a walker in front of them for a brace point.

Sitting down is similar

1. Make sure the chair/ bed is locked and secured
2. Back up until they feel the bed/chair behind their legs.
3. Leaning SLIGHTLY forward (Yell, "Timber," just kidding.)
4. Squat until in a full sitting position.

Level Two

Little more work.

From bed to chair, they need to sit, with a gait belt around them and shoes on. Plan your task accordingly, giving yourself a step-by-step checklist.

Know your landing point and how far you need to go to be there.

1. Stand with feet shoulder length apart, brace your Loved One under the arms and hold the belt near the back sides at kidney level.
2. Keeping your back straight and your knee touching theirs.
3. Straddle the weaker leg of theirs, bend at the hips, and stand up straight bringing your Loved One with you.
4. Stand tall and pause for steadiness before moving again.
5. Two-Step sway dance works great as you turn to set them down (for ambulation farther than right here, see different types to ambulate).
6. Project their landing and adjust the angle before making contact.
7. Check for any discomfort after landing has been made.

*TIP: Counting to three while rocking will give momentum to stand on three.

The closer the locations, the better. Strive for it. YEAH!!!!!

Level Three

Now, this one is tricky, tricky, tricky.

You have a few options to help you. A gait belt is a must for this one.

Transferring by yourself:

1. Apply the gait belt and prepare the chair right next to the bed, locking and securing it for a 90-degree angle pivot turn. The front of the chair should be a couple of inches from your Loved One's closest leg.

2. Take the leg closest to the chair, cross that foot over the other and away from the chair.

3. Straddle their legs.

4. Bend at the hips and straighten your back. Hold on tight and rock, lift with your knees and pull them up on the count of three.

5. At this level there may not be time to stand fully erect. Step with free leg towards the chair and pivot turn, lowering them into the chair.

6. This also works in reverse (chair to bed).

7. Just make sure the direction you are going, have the closest foot crossed over and brace with the farthest knee. Please keep in mind the power of weight throwing and your precious back.

The sidekick saves you in that department. I forgot to tell you, you might need to go and get a back brace. This duty can take a toll on your body the more you must do for your Loved One.

Transferring with a sidekick:

1. Have each of you standing on the opposing side of your Loved One.

2. Using the arms farthest from your Loved One, reach around and grab the belt in the backside. And with the arm closest to your Loved One, lock arms at the elbows.

3. Bracing knee to knee closest to you and your sidekick as your reflection, rock and lift on the count of three.

4. Stand and step to pivot. Gently lower them into the chair that you have previously placed and locked into position.

This also works in reverse (chair to bed).

Your sidekick may not be able to fit in the threshold area should it be a small room so they may need to alter their position to accommodate the environment.

*TIP: A slide board is used like a conveyer belt.

If your Loved One's weight is an issue, I feel it's best to do it with a slide board.

Using a Slide Board

1. Loved One is sitting on the bed with the draw sheet under them. Place the wheelchair next to them and lock the wheels. Pull the side arm of the chair closest to the bed up and to the back.

2. Lift the sheet (side between your Loved One and the chair) and slide the board underneath as far as to know it is stable, leaving the board to bridge the gap between the bed and the chair. Make sure they are going to be pulled towards you.

3. Make sure the bed is <u>slightly</u> higher than the chair so we use gravity.

4. Along with bracing the board, hold the sheet and slowly slide them downhill into the chair. Pull until they are fully in the chair.

5. While holding the sheet, grab the gait with the other hand and pull towards you to complete the slide. This is centering their whole butt in the chair.

6. Lift the sheet from under them and pull the board out.

7. Drape the visible sheets over your Loved One's lap and lock the armrest back in place. To hide the sheet, roll and tuck on the sides.

8. Please don't forget to buckle any safety restraints and put their feet on the foot pedals.

Hoyer Lift

The Hoyer Life is mainly for a Loved One who is non-weight bearing and is too heavy to move on your own or with someone. It is also the one thing mandatory for two people to assist. And yes, I know you may not have help, but if you can, please get an extra set of hands. Otherwise, you can only do as best as you can. I strongly recommend having an extra set of hands for the controls, but if you have to do it by yourself, so be it. Or better yet, don't do it. But if you must, practice with a heavy object first. Practice and practice until you are ready for the real thing. You do not want to have someone fall out.

1. Make sure the sling is right side up and not backward or inside out. The handles in the back are on the outside and the hole is where the butt goes if it has it. There are other types of slings. Please request a tutorial on those specific ones.

    2.   Lay the sling over your Loved One to generalize placement. Ensure the sling reaches only down to just below the back of their knees. Bend the knee to see if the sling is still touching the back of the knees. If it's not, move it down until it does while bent.

    3.   Roll it towards you halfway and your Loved One away from you. Place rolled up half under them until you can't see the rolled part. Roll them back to you and hold them up while you roll the sling back out behind them.

    4.   Double-checking alignments at this time will let you make adjustments before it's too late. I might say that a lot. AKA. Repeat! Both sides are even.

    5.   Please make sure the sling reaches the back of the head or higher but still just below the knee.

    6.   Scan for obstructions in pathway and underneath the bed such as electronic cords, tubing, etc.

    7.   Raise the height of the bed and lower the railings.

    8.   Position the Hoyer Lift over your Loved One and lock the wheels.

    9.   Position hooks close to the chest.

    10.   Match the colors per side. Head = same color / Feet = same color. The color closest to the sling makes that side higher.

    11.   You can angle what color to use according to how high you need them to sit and how far back you want them in the chair. On the top is usually the first color and the bottom is one color or two colors away.

    12.   When they are hooked, double-check.

13. Double check pathway and no tubes connecting your Loved One to the bed. If tubing is attached, put those connected things on their lap.

14. Make sure the chair is either against the wall or locked to keep the chair from moving.

15. Raise the arm claw enough to see tightness. Stop.

16. Triple-check that the straps are still hooked correctly. Continue to go up.

17. Only go up enough to clear all obstacles and is able to float over the bed.

18. Pull out and away from the bed and turn towards chair. You can come in diagonally over the chair, but no wall should be behind it. The wall may prevent the legs from being in the proper position.

19. Legs open wider with a lever and make it fit on the outside of wheels.

20. Turn the sling where your Loved One is parallel over the chair (facing you) and lock the Hoyer wheels.

21. Pushing on their knees so they land farther back in the chair with the other hand releasing them down slowly.

22. Should it not align the first time, lift them up and try again. I'd say after the third try, you're done. Carefully put them back in the bed and try again later.

23. This also works in reverse as well (to the bed).

Being in a sling can cause a lot of anxiety for your Loved One so the less time in the sling, the better the stress levels.

*** TIP:** Check, Check, and Recheck. Being absolutely positive is key.

Assist Devices

Security bars are the best for your Loved One to hold on to while adjusting, dressing, etc. Least dangerous with the wheelchair locked and behind them, should their knees buckle and they go down. Normally people at Levels One and Two use walkers for transfer. Just help brace the walker so it is more stable for them.

Chapter 7: Ambulation

To transport your Loved One from one location to another. This is the dance of all dances to glide across the room and soar through worlds to another location altogether. Not only is this exercise for you, but it is freeing for your Loved One. Both Benefit. BOOM!

I know this section is pretty short but the main thing for you to know is the two of you need to cooperate with each other to have a safe ambulation. Safety above all.

*TIP: Always support their weaker side for ambulation and keep an eye on them leaning to one side more than the other.

Wheelchair

This is self-explanatory. Keep in mind your path and terrain. Never take the road less traveled unless they are completely independent and even then, it is risky.

When pushing a wheelchair, think of it as a dolly carrying a fragile and priceless case of crystal glass. How you move with a moving dolly is kind of the same way. You can't push uphill, you need to take them up tilted backward and if real steep, a second person to follow up will help secure safe travel.

On a flat surface, you should be on all four wheels. No wheelies. If the path is narrow, there is no turning around. Back out the way you came in.

Same for going downhill, just in reverse. Going downhill means you'll go down facing forward, tilting back. Handicap ramps, you can go face ahead because steepness is low. You can only really ambulate two different ways; walking or wheeling.

***TIP:** Keeping their feet up on foot pedals will ensure you don't wheel over their feet and legs and they don't fall or slide out. It is also considered a brace point for your Loved One and a sense of control for them to hold their body in the chair if no safety restraint is available.

Walker

Walking is guided with a walker and security belt. When walking, ensure they stand tall and keep the walker close to them. No reaching and bent backs. It shouldn't be strenuous.

Make sure the walker's height matches the length of the arm reach for your Loved One, who is standing straight up. It can be adjusted on the legs and make sure all four legs are even.

Walking

Life moves fast when you are mobile, so, please keep your Loved One intact and all attachments attached and safe. If needed, there should be a place on the walker and wheelchair to hang attached devices. For catheters, there should be something like a cloth bag that we call a dignity bag. If you don't have one, make one. Just get a good bag and put a metal hook on it so it can hang freely and discreetly.

Ways to walk

- Dance Walking - to music or even humming a tune.
- Mirrored Walking - when you step, they step.
- Counting Walking - every count to a step or left/right repeat.

These all help people who forget to walk the way they are used to. Don't be mad at them. Help them.

DON'T

Hoyer Lift is only a transfer device, NOT an ambulation device or substitute for a wheelchair. The probability of falling is high because they swing as you move.

Chapter 8: Range of Motion & Occupational Therapy

Range of Motion (ROM)

Something in motion stays in motion. That's why we walk, stretch, and exercise. For your Loved One, there is no exception. They should do the same or they will stiffen like the tinman. Keep them oiled by doing exercises and stretches. Occupational Therapy helps with their independence and everyday living.

We don't know how much ROM your Loved One is able to do, but we should still try so that they do not stiffen. So, if it seems too much, break it up through the day for some and through the week for others. You can even make your own exercise regiment, but nothing extreme. Listen to them and go slow because you don't want them to break or tear anything.

IN THE BED

(DO NOT FORCE THESE EXERCISES) Always support the limb exercising.

1. Doing them in the bed is the most beneficial for you both. It helps you physically and contains any accidents that may occur. Laying in the bed and bending the knees, push the pelvis to the ceiling and take the butt completely off the bed. This helps with the back, core, legs and butt muscles. Keeps everything strong. You can even do these for yourself. Work out together. This is for people who are able to do it, not everyone can, so be sure to not force the exercise.

2. Keeping the knees bent, lean the knees from side to side. You'll feel it in the hips. Good stretch.

3. Showgirl leg-kicks from a bent or straight leg position. Now don't go crazy and hyper-extend anything. This is purely a limitation stretch, not FULL HIGH KICKS.

4. Hamstring stretches with high knees to the chest. If you can, hold for 3 seconds and release slowly.

5. Dancers' feet - point feet like a ballerina, flex, and try to look under your toes.

6. Rolling ankles. Both directions.

Here are some additional ROM stretches that can be done anywhere. This is not a full list, but should encompass the main parts of the body. Always have your Loved One in a stable position hanging onto a wall, sofa, or device if they're not able to balance properly. Always follow the directions of your Physical Therapist.

1. Head and Neck - tilt head from left to right and front to back, look left to right, and roll head in a circle from left to right and right to left

2. Spine – bend over knees to try to touch toes being careful so as not to fall forward, lean from side to side trying to touch the floor, lean side to side with arms in the air 'reaching for the sky'

3. Shoulders – should lifts raising your shoulders like a shrug

4. Shoulder Circles – roll shoulders in a circle

5. Arms – a windmill motion front to back and back to front

6. Wrist – wrist turns rolling them from side to side or in a circle

7. Fingers – spread fingers apart and then ball them into a fist

8. Thumb – stretch thumb backwards and forwards and then rotate in a circle

9. Hip – move leg out to the side and then bring back in front crossing other leg

10. Knees – bending the leg at the knee trying to touch rear
11. Calf – sitting down, lift heels off of floor
12. Ankles – roll ankle in a circle, flex up and down like a ballerina
13. Toes – wiggle toes and spread away from each other

These you and your Loved One may or may not be able to do and that's okay. The goal is to get there. Overdoing is not our goal. It gives them a slew of choice exercises that stimulate the body. You can also do these exercises in the sitting position and incorporate furniture, such as a chair while doing butt lifts, for example. This will work other muscles, such as arms in their entirety, pectoral muscles, and even the back. If you can, make it a game like SIMON SAYS. That is the most fun, especially with a group of people such as your family.

Again, have fun, but don't overdo it.

Occupational Therapy (OT)

Occupational Therapy is when your Loved One is getting ready for the day or trying to get back into a routine of how to do something. This is also called Active Daily Living (ADL). It is getting them back to normal or as close as you can by exercising the actions taken to care for oneself, like getting dressed, cleaning, eating, balancing, etc. For my grandfather, he goes to check the mail. This is considered a routine for his daily activities. Having them do more for themselves activates their occupational skills of living. Don't neglect them. If they can't do it, help them, but if they can, promote that independence they so rightfully have and desire. When people do it for themselves, it feels so good that they just might keep it up and do more. Although we are still aging, don't stunt anyone's growth.

Now, let's talk about the next few chapters and the literal mess that is to come. Warning: the literal poo in your life from now on.

***FRUIT: You don't know how appreciated it is until you are the one doing the appreciating.**

Throughout our lives, we are CONTINENT. That is, we are able to hold our bladder and bowels until we get to the bathroom. We were potty trained at a very young age and we practice this our whole lives.

As we get older, we tend to become SEMI-INCONTINENT or unable to hold it sometimes. This is when our bladder muscles give a little leeway and leaking occurs.

At some point, we will end up INCONTINENT which means we can't hold it ever. What we trained ourselves to work for us is now something we must work around.

When you're unable to use the toilet, this is when you're forced to go in the bed. We spend our whole lives trying not to do that, only to turn around and have to. Confusing but necessary. It takes a big hit to your Loved One's dignity to ask for help with something that they have done for themselves their whole lives. Modesty goes right out the window in situations like these and please keep your feelings to yourself. You are going to smell something you don't like and please keep the gagging down to barely spotted. Embarrassment is hard to overcome and I don't want you to taint their only source to help them. Some people have too much pride to ask for help and will go without cleansing if they can't do it alone.

Chapter 9: But First Let Me Brief You

This tells you the styles of underwear you are going to encounter and how to use them. This chapter should help you decipher which item is easier to use and possible alterations you can make to best fit your Loved One. You'll also find alternative uses for the extra items you no longer use regularly.

I'll make you an easy guide to the type of underwear you are going to encounter.

Regular Underwear (Self-explanatory)	Doesn't stretch as well, needs to undress.	Fully change if soiled
Disposable Underwear (Pull-ups)	Stretches great, easy to manipulate.	Easy to rip the side open and off
Brief with tabs (Adult Diaper)	You don't have to undress really.	Tabs that are detachable

UNDERWEAR

Not much to say about the already known. Underwear is underwear. However, you do need to get the right size to fit. Too loose can fall off and too tight can cause abrasions around our natural creases in the groin area. The too big will not hold any extra absorbent item in place.

PADS

All women and maybe most, if not ALL men, know what pads are. However, what people don't know is there are also pads in the triangle shape fit for men. Yes, men have incontinent issues too. Read the direction of which way is the front. Some have a wider spot, usually the front.

If pads are not enough, people usually move on to:

PULL-UPS

These are disposable underwear that are supposed to tear easily on the side, but some may need scissors. Some have colored tag indicators for the back, yet some will be floral on the front for design. Some, you can see the wider side be the indicator for the bum-bum. Some people use pads along with pull-ups. Make sure placement is between center to front for men and dead center for women. Placement is key in order to get full use out of them.

BRIEFS

Adult diaper with tabs to hold together. Its shape is not accurate to form fit for our bodies and you can always alter with scissors. Make sure not to cut the tab's connection, you will render it useless. And try to stay away from the padded part. It is a cotton like substance inside that when wet, it turns into a jelly like material which can be really messy to clean up.

WASHABLE PAD

These types of pads are washable as opposed to disposable (see CHUCKS below). They are the least expensive route because they are reusable. These should be washed after every soiling and it's best to have two or more for easy changeout.

CHUCKS AKA CHUX

Disposable under pads that you can pretty much put anywhere to protect everything your Loved One sits or lays on. Don't treat your Loved One as contaminated, be gentle with your words. We call these chucks because, when you're done with it, you chuck it.

MAKE-SHIFT PADS

If push comes to shove and you don't have any of the above, other absorbent disposable items can be used, such as paper towels, cut up disposable under pads, or even baby diapers as long as they do not cause any irritation to the area.

My dear friend Candy was able to use a baby diaper as a wraparound pad catching all urine for her late husband. It was a diaper within a diaper. She put the box within the box. I love her. This saved them from having to change him so often.

If underwear is frequently checked, you can swap out the smaller diaper for a dry one and prolong the clean life of that underwear. You can also use any extra pull-ups as pads if your Loved One has graduated to briefs. Trim around the pad, making it a bigger pad. This, too, can also be slid out and replaced, prolonging the life of the brief.

MAKE-SHIFT CHUCKS AKA CHUX

Along with a towel, garbage bags are your best friend in times of need. Open the garbage bag by making a rectangle, laying it down first and then lay a towel on top. Make sure the plastic is covered wherever your Loved One is going to touch. BOOM!

See what else you can use to makeshift all that you may be lacking.

I dare you.

Chapter 10: Checks and Changes

Do you pee? How about Poop? If you said yes, that's great. So does your Loved One, probably more than you do. Or at least it's more noticeable only because they rely on you to help them. Now, if you are not too keen on helping someone use the bathroom, you had better get over it real fast because this is where most of your action is all day. Frequently going to the restroom is what we do subconsciously, so it must be available for them.

Checks and changes keep our Loved Ones feeling dry, clean, and comfortable. It's important to find out what kind of check schedule you need to keep up with your changing of linen to reduce your laundry loads.

Checks

Every time you check your Loved One's continent status, you prolong the life of the underwear type they are wearing. This is important since it will save you and your Loved One many disruptions throughout the day.

Determine a Check Schedule:

A full day is twenty-four hours. You should check and prepare to change them every four hours. If their linens are soiled within four hours of prior check time, your Loved One has one of the good bladders (in a professional's eyes) and needs to be checked more frequently. Set your alarm. Charting the bathroom times and comparing over a few days, you should be able to map out a generalized time frame of when your Loved One needs to be changed regularly. A portion of this can be prevented by changing one to two times throughout the night and following when they get up in the morning.

Depending on the level of peeing they do, only changing them once a day is a form of neglect especially if the skin starts to break down. You need to keep their skin dry and change them often, paying attention to more soiled areas and how the pee looks when not changed.

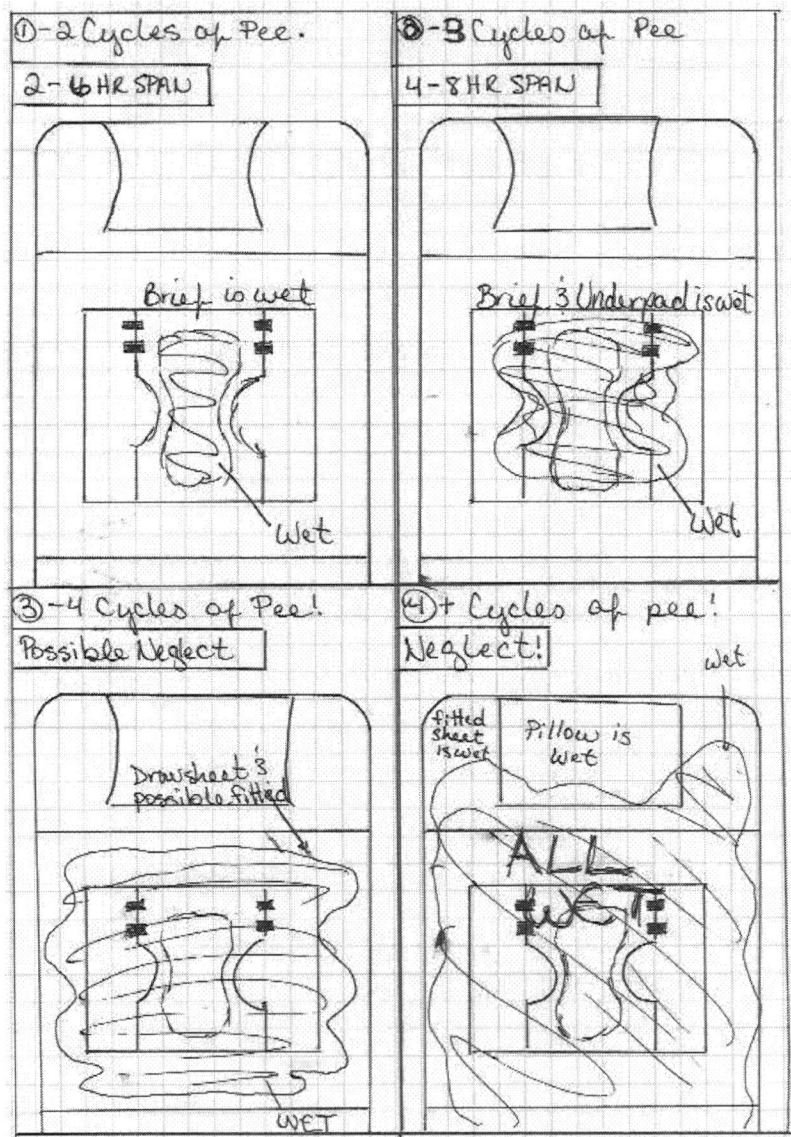

Preparation is KEY

If an accident occurs, Change and Replace.

Depending on how soiled you find your Loved One, you will have laundry duty following you. It can be anywhere from just the underwear or the whole bed. Remember, less will need to be changed and replaced if checked frequently. Always ask if they need to use the restroom, depending on their capability.

Prepare for your changing task and retrieve everything required before you start.

1. Gloves
2. Wash basin with warm water, or as hot as they like
4. Washcloth
5. Medium towel
6. Wipes
7. Protective barrier creme
8. Linens and protective pad to keep underneath them.

Pre-maid Linen Roll

What is a premade roll, you ask? It consists of what should be on the bed, under your Loved One, all the way to their skin. This is for a brief.

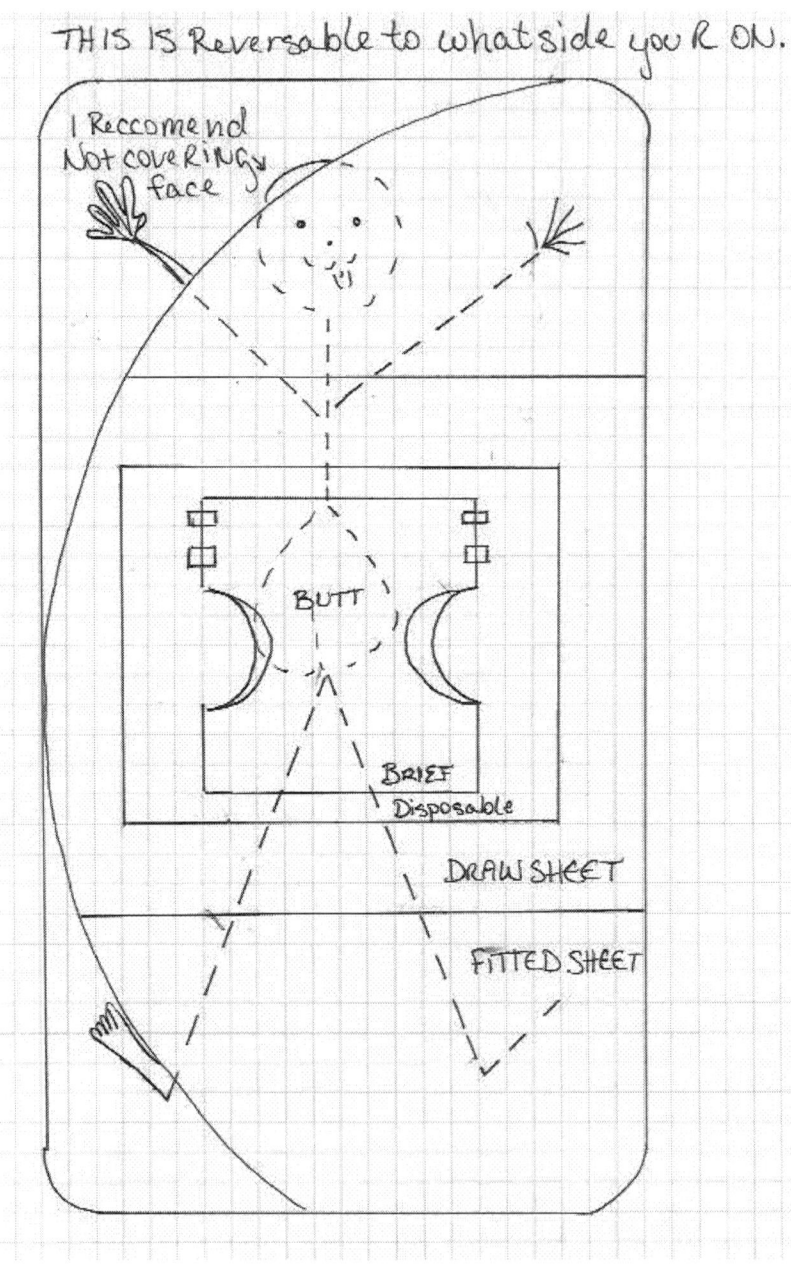

- 1st. Fitted Sheet (the very bottom)
- 2nd. Disposable Chuck *upside down (optional for easy slide)
- 3rd. Draw Sheet
- 4th. Disposable Chuck *right side up
- 5th. Brief (last on top) completely open

Then your Loved One goes on top of all that.

- Roll towards you halfway so it will mirror your Loved One's behind and land dead center.

See how far down this list is soiled and replace what's needed.

A premade linen roll containing all the linen needed to be changed in order as above. Place where you feel will fit your Loved Ones best, on top of each other, rolling everything towards you.

Wah-La! Premade roll. This keeps you from rolling your Loved One more than once and causing more discomfort.

*TIP: Doubling up on the pads and placing the extra chucks staggered one over the other under your Loved One at night will help if they're a heavy wetter.

For level 1 or 2, move them out of bed and somewhere safe while you make the bed. For level 3, you will have to change the bed with them in it.

A tabbed brief can be incorporated into your premade. Underwear and Pull-ups, you can pull up as far as you can before rolling them over to pull it up in the back. Be careful if you use the method of having them lift their butt. It can roll up their skin in the back so please look out and make sure it is smooth underneath.

Changing "Underwear" In the Bedroom.

Level One

1. Depending on how soaked they are and their abilities, take them to the shower to rinse and wash their body from the breast and back all the way down. Like a semi-shower.

2. To do a basic linen change, change their underwear and or brief with them standing up. Pull down their underwear and change. Simple.

   a. If long-term stability is limited, have them sit down on a chuck after they have pulled down their soiled garments. They can hold a walker to stand while you clean them, or they can roll over on the bed to reach the backside.
   b. After doing so, dress them in the new underwear and pad/or brief.
   c. Tabs are in the back and wrap around to the front for a brief and designs goes in the front for a pull-up.

3. For a Pull-up
   a. If they're in a standing position, pull it up all the way, otherwise pull it up as far as it goes making sure it didn't roll down anywhere. If they are laying down, turn them on their side and pull it up in the back and do it again on the reverse side.
   b. Make sure the bottom lining of the pad is centered and the sides are in the natural creases of the groin.

Level Two

This s similar to level one but may be more debilitating since they need more of your help. Be gentler with their joints while rolling or sitting/standing. Hold them near and steadier with one hand while you dress them with the other.

Level Three

Bedbound Loved Ones are different since they will have more steps to follow. Please, I beg you, if your Loved One needs to use the restroom, a bedside commode is best because they are of NO help to you in a tight restroom. Being near the bed would fit best for safety reasons, okay?!

* **Tip:** The more frequently you check, the less you need to change. And guess what! Less laundry. Remember a changing chart helps figure out what your Loved Ones' bathroom schedule is like.

Changing Them in the Bed

1. Undress your Loved One mid-drift only. No one gets fully naked to go to the bathroom. Well, there might be some. Cover them with a towel.
2. Tuck all the soiled linen far under your Loved One, on the opposite side that you are working from.
3. Always make the side of the bed that you are on and lay it over your Loved One, removing wrinkles and straightening it out.
4. Make sure the back of the brief is high enough to meet their belly button, but no higher. This will help ensure their entire bottom is covered.

5. Roll all the clean linen to you and tucked between the side of the bed and your body.

6. Wet wipes in the basin with water and no-rinse wash. Ring out lightly and drench the front. Cleaning the front down to the back, leave the soiled wipes underneath that crevice. Repeat until the front has no visible poo and/or is washed clean of pee.

For Females: Wipe clean to dirty, leave the wipe in the soiled brief underneath near the rear. Never go back up with wipes. Get a new one. Spread the lips apart, clean in and scoop down and OUT, always going in a down and away motion.

For Males: Wipe clean to dirty, starting at the tip, go down the shaft between the creases and push down into the soiled brief. If they still have their foreskin, pull it back and clean thoroughly. Infections are riskier with foreskin.

7. Push soiled brief down between their legs towards their backside.

8. Rinse well.

9. After area is clean and no visible soil is present wash and rinse over again with a washcloth.

10. Dry thoroughly

11. If cream is used, generously cover external area avoiding any entrances as it can burn if it gets inside (should be for topical external use only).

12. Recover with a towel

13. Roll your Loved One from you, so you may pull out the dirty linen.

14. Tuck your premade roll under their visible back facing you. Make sure you pull their skin up and out of the way while the other hand pushes the premade roll down and into the bed under their skin.

15. Roll them away from you, but be sure you don't roll them off the bed. Put a pillow where they should land and rest. If in a hospital bed, put it against the railing and have them hold on. This keeps them from smashing their face against the bar.

16. Slowly pull (no rips) the soiled out, but leave it under just enough to catch any excrement collected below. Clean the soiled backside with wipes first, leaving them on the soiled pile, pulled away from the body.

17. Take the soiled pile and roll it up like a sub sandwich and discard. Sorry, I didn't mean to ruin lunch for you. LOL (Loved One Laughing).

18. Use the washcloth and dry with a towel. Set them aside to put in laundry once the mission is completed.

19. Now, take your new premade roll and place it precisely under your Loved One (still rolled on their side). Mirroring the body and where it would fit, eyeball the landing of their bottom, being perfectly centered in the middle of it. Now it is not supposed to be fully rolled out yet.

20. Stuff the roll far enough under them while picking up the skin to keep from pinching.

21. Apply barrier cream to the bottom before turning them back to you.

22. Before rolling the other side out, make sure the tabbed side looks right for an accurate landing of coverage, or you will have to readjust it.

23. When you see or feel the premade roll on the other side, roll it out completely, looking for the other end of every new piece of linen replaced. If you don't see it, you may need them to lean the other way to help find it.

24. Pull the front of the brief through their slightly spread legs.

25. Pull the legs slightly apart, not enough to hurt, but to ensure the brief doesn't cut into the fatty part of their thighs. If it does, after a while, it becomes a rash, so watch their leg fat. The brief should fit in the NATURAL crease in the groin. Not one you made. Fasten the tabs and call it a day!

26. Stretch the brief out a little for the natural creases. If it is too tight, it can start a rash or tear the skin and have a sore begin.

27. Complete the bed making and pull on the sheets to straighten underneath them to keep them wrinkle free.

***TIP:** I know you may not get it right the first time, but you will have plenty of time to practice for perfection. Oh yeah! Don't forget to ensure the brief end (with tabs) is on their backside, not frontside, nor too far up their back. You have less in the front to tab on.

If there is no accident, and they would like to sit on the toilet....

Chapter 11: To The Toilet!

Toileting is something that is going to occur the most throughout the day. Sometimes it is "Easy-Peasy," and sometimes, it's not.

Preparation is KEY

Know what you need and the location you are going to. Having a routine location like the bathroom and an emergency location like the bedside commode, depending on how big of the urgency, you need to know how to undress them with quickness and yet gently. Already knowing how to transfer, this will become a piece of cake (chocolate).

Again, know your plan and the tools you need before performing your duties.

Level one

1. Take them to the bathroom and let them use the toilet. While they are sitting on the toilet, look at their underwear, is it dirty? If it is, completely remove the pants with underwear and replace the soiled ones. If it's a pull-up, rip or cut the sides of the pull-up and pull it out through the legs, rolling it up and putting it in the trash.

2. If you pull down their pull-up and oops, there's poo bear, cut or rip the sides and tug the pull-up through to the back wiping up the crack with the remaining clean part. Roll it up before throwing it in the trash. Let them sit down on the toilet and if they are not done, let them finish, then help them wipe clean and sit back down.

3. Putting a new pull-up on requires only undressing one leg. Apply the pull-up and bring it up to the thighs, then return the naked leg back to the pant owner and empty the pant leg.

4. If you are out and your Loved One is shy about getting undressed, put the pull-up on one foot, feeding it through the pant leg to the top and then feeding it back down the other pant leg to the foot, sliding foot in pull-up hole. Then pull them up like underwear. Don't pull too hard on the pull-up as it can tear easily. This method is questionable depending on the clothes restriction and excessive weight.

5. If getting up and down is hard, after they do their biz, keep them sitting down and put the new pull-up on before standing to wipe.

*TIP: Put a temporary disposable paper towel of some sort between their legs, covering the new pull-up underneath. This will prevent any after-leakage or additional accident resulting in changing the pull-up again. Been there, done that, bought the T-Shirt and scrapbooked it.

6. If they use a walker, the process would be the same, but you will have to work around the walker and keep it in front of them for stability. Still holding that gait belt. Safety first!

7. Wiping them may seem hard, but please remember, if you hold the gait belt up higher than their waist, feel some weight of your Loved One. You will feel the weight change and prepare to lower them back on the toilet as slowly as you can, should they start to fall.

Now remember, as a PROUD SOILED LINEN, your safety is important to remember so you may carry the weight of others. So, your stance is very important and to hold your feet at shoulder length apart, with the foot farther from the toilet, close to the knee, for further guidance back onto the toilet if a fall should occur.

8.   You will be facing the profile of your Loved One. While holding the gait belt in the front and wiping with the hand closest to the butt. The tub on one side, Soiled Linen (you) on the other.

9.   If the bathroom is just a toilet room, grab bars are going to be very necessary. If the wheelchair fits, you probably won't. Make sure your Loved One is able to move properly before putting them in a predicament in such a small space.

10.   If the bathroom is too small or you don't have any room, you can have them stand up and put their hands on the wall. Tell them, "Freeze! Put your hands up!" Then they are holding themselves up with the wall while your hands dress your Loved One. Be aware that your Loved One's legs can buckle and fall to the floor, So I suggest using a gait belt and standing with one of your legs in between theirs. I don't want to get off the subject, so to know what a gait belt is, refer back to *Repositioning, Transfers, and Ambulation*.

Level Two

If your Loved One cannot stand on their own, but can transfer from chair to toilet, chances are they can hold themselves up with the wall technique while you finish dressing them. Putting the bedside commode on top of the toilet also helps with stability because now they have side handles to help them stand or sit. Even a toilet riser with handles does the same.

1.   With one of my ladies, I always say, "Stand tall, hands to wall." And she holds herself up while I dress her.

*TIP: Now, don't get short with them if they can't stand and dress. People sometimes need to focus more on the task and less on stability so their equilibrium sometimes goes off-kilter. This is where you hold their stability for them.

    2.   So, sit down. Vertigo is no joke.

    3.   If not, they can hold on to you while you hold them up with one hand and dress them with the other hand. Please use the handlebars.

*TIP: Feeling the stability in your poised posture and strong like a cement pillar gives them confidence in your decisions and they will follow your lead. No spaghetti arms.

Level Three

To the Bedside Commode – in the Bedroom

Usually, you will not have a pull-up on your Loved One if they are bedbound. It is more efficient and cleaner to be able to see under them versus feeling your way while holding them up. More than likely, they will be in a brief where you can undo the side tabs before transferring. If they are wearing a pull-up, rip the sides, push the dirty down and away so you don't bring it with you onto the toilet.

Now you can do this in two different ways.

    1.   If you have a bedside commode that is placed near the lower side of the bed facing the headboard, your Loved One can transfer, with your help, safely to the commode and give them privacy to do their biz.

    * Tip: Line the commode bucket with a waste basket-sized bag or grocery bag. Check for holes, please, or it's a whole other mess you will have to clean up. Putting a Clorox wipe or paper towel with vinegar and water in the bottom will keep the smell down and make it easier to clean.

2. Using the bedside commode over the toilet - undress the bottom half first

Taking a Level Three Loved One to the toilet in the bathroom is very difficult to do and hard to clean vital places. So, I only suggest this if they are going into the shower right after. You can use the bedside commode as a shower chair, but remember to remove the collection bucket first, and place the bucket on the floor underneath the chair.

So, let's just do a safe play, use the bedside commode, and call it a day, okay?

Look at me! Ghostwriter for rappers, say what?!

If your Loved One is already soiled and you just find out as you are putting them on the toilet, you have a few more steps added ahead for you. They are still dressed.

No Bedside Commode – to the Toilet

For the Brief

1. First, you pull your Loved One (in the wheelchair) close to the toilet. Ask them to lift up a little so you can slide their pants down to their knees.

2. This should reveal the tabs of the brief. If they can't help you, you're going to have to suck it up and put your muscle shirt on. Kind of wiggle the pants down to the knees. Granted, you might end up sliding your Loved One down in the chair so, you're going to push the same knee of the side you're pulling down.

3. Alternate back and forth until the pants slide the rest of the way easily.

4. If you have already slid them down to the point they are going to fall out and the gait belt doesn't help or is absent at the time, go around to the back and hug them from behind. Grab their forearms from under their arms, tell them to hold you close and pull them up in the chair. Go back to the front and continue undressing.

5. If your Loved One slides down and there are two people available, have them stand on the side opposite of you facing your Loved One and putting their arm closest to them and with the other hand (farther away) grab their pants and lift together ON three. They should be back in the chair. Continue to undress them to the knees.

6. Undo the tabs and pull the tabs to the back and off their body. Take the front of the brief and pull down as you pull up one leg at a time, ensuring it's completely under their legs and not stuck between them. We don't want it to go with your Loved One on or in the toilet. If you did it right, it would be in the wheelchair or on the floor. Hopefully, not on the floor because that will give you a couple of other steps called "Cleaning the floor and whatever else it touched."

7. To make sure they are clean, you'll need them to lean as far forward without falling off so you can reach the back to clean. I usually stand halfway in front and halfway on the side as they hug your waist for stability. Gloves would be a great idea, ok? In fact, at all changes and cleanings.

8. Put the clean brief in the chair open for your Loved One to sit on. Taking the tabs out to the side so they aren't stuck behind them when they sit. Transfer them back into the chair on top of the brief. Pull the front of the brief up between their legs, making sure you don't catch any of their thigh fat in the brief.

9. Open it to latch with the tabs. Pull their pants up as far as you can before you try to have them stand then pull up their pants the rest of the way. Let them plop back in their seat because they will be pooped. No pun intended.

For the Pull-Up

1 Rip the sides and lift your Loved One straight up and on to the toilet.

2 Throw the pull-up away that was left in the chair.

3 After they finish, begin to wipe them up as best as you can.

4 With a clean chuck in the chair, pick your Loved One up and sit them on top of the chair.

5 Wheel them back into the room, where they can lay on the bed while you make sure they are thoroughly clean.

6 Apply the new pull-up and put their pants back on.

7 Dress them when you are done and clean up the mess.

If the pants aren't wet, put them back on. If they are, change them. Ensure the whole soiled area is washed and dry before dressing.

Brief change for someone who wants to use the toilet is sometimes tricky for a Level Three Loved One. Briefs might be better to change than a pull-up if you can't hold them up and dress them simultaneously. I know, discombobulating. If you can hold them up with your leg while they hold onto a wall, you don't need to fully undress the bottom, just push down the pants to the knees and work the brief between the legs. Pull the tabbed sides around your Loved One (kind of like a hug from behind) and tab in the front of the brief where both will meet.

Chapter 12: Oops… There's Poo!

The importance of your Loved One's poo:

It is the collection of what's in your body and as it comes out you will find out that it's telling on your Loved One internally. They may look fine from the outside; however, the waste will tell you otherwise.

Poo and his friend, Urinella, are only looking out for the best of your Loved One by eliminating the body's trash (stuff, it doesn't need or want). However, it can only eliminate so much because the body takes in the good and accidentally brings some bad and has damage after. This is why it is important to only fill or fuel with things that are good for you. Flushing with water is the best and the most needed for your body.

Urinella

Urinella likes to play the game "Show and Tell" with color and clarity. From clear to cloudy, it will determine kidney or urinary tract issues.

1. From CLEAR to LIGHT YELLOW means it is normal and healthy.
2. DARK YELLOW means dehydration and you need to flush your system with more water throughout the day.
3. ORANGE and BROWN can mean liver issues and need attention if it doesn't subside with flushing of water daily.
4. RED means blood or prostate issues.
5. FOAMY or CLOUDY thick-looking urine is issues with the kidneys or excess protein.
6. Other colors can be food dyes in drinks.

See a doctor if there's any worries about the color or consistency of the urine or if any pain is coming from your Loved One while urinating. Keep in mind that your Loved One may not feel any pain yet still have a urinary tract infection (UTI).

Looks like Poo, Smells like Poo, Must be Poo. Don't Taste It.

Poo likes to play too, showing color and consistency:

1. Any shade in BROWN means it's normal.

2. Any shade in GREEN means you have been eating a lot of greens or have a possible bacterial infection.

3. Any shade of YELLOW means liver condition or lack of bile.

4. Any shade of RED means possible new blood from damage like hemorrhoids or internal bleeding. It varies.

5. Any shade of BLACK means possible excess of iron or "old" blood coming from the upper G.I. tract.

6. Any shade of WHITE means possible pre-existing medical condition or issue with bile workings.

IN OTHER NEWS, food dyes can also do this to your poo, so consider what you ate and if you are still leery, please see your doctor.

Consistency for Poo

1. Liquid poo with no solid means inflammation and possible dehydration.

2. Mush means inflammation.

3. Soft blobs broken apart means a lack of fiber.

4. Like a smooth snake means normal.

5. Sausage holding itself together as much as possible means normal.

6. Candy Bar might be a sign of constipation.

7. Hard Deer Pellets mean constipation.

All of these must be monitored and if it persists after every attempt in fixing, go to the DOCTOR!

The major way to attract any and everything is through poo. Constipation is the sheets and hurts as well. Be compassionate about your Loved One's emotions during this tough time. Constipation causes irritation because it feels like you are on the verge of going to the bathroom, but it just won't come out.

A slew of things can help with constipation. Let's start from the least invasive.

1. Natural, Over the Counter, or Prescribed Medicines

Anything from prune juice to Milk of Magnesium to medications.

Start with something natural like prune juice. This usually does the trick, but watch it! God's creation is powerful, so is coconut and pineapple. Bananas make me go too, but consider the potassium intake and consult the doctor about how many bananas is the limit per day for this.

2. Needing Assistance (Sometimes we all need a little help)

Physical stimulation - I'm talking about coaching the poo out. Pushing on the sides of the rectum will help form the poo on the inside to make its way out smoothly. Don't push too hard, you can hurt them and they may never let you down there again. Then they will try to do it themselves and then you have a worse scenario.

Enema – Be careful because it can explode in your face. It's not really like that, but when you are dealing with it at the time, it does feel that way. So, stay calm but try to be quick to catch it. Not with your hands. The nearest thing you're not afraid to get dirty that can spread open to catch the explosive aftermath.

Giving an Enema

Level One

Having your Loved One lay down on their side and then being able to make it to the toilet is risky, but possible. More likely, having any protective guard down and a very close range to the toilet are major factors of successful hygienic execution and clean result, leaving the dignity and comfort levels untouched and heightened. You can also insert the enema while they are on the toilet. Just have them lean as far forward for you to see what you are doing and make sure you insert at the same angle as their rectum is facing.

Level Two

These Loved Ones know what they would like to do, as opposed to what they can do. Your level of ability to stabilize your Loved One will determine what is safe for them and the best route for the execution of the task.

Staying in a lying position after insertion and pooping is probable and an easier task for many reasons, but one thing for sure, no falling down in a mess of poo. This is less transferring with depleted energy and easier to contain the mess.

Level Three

You would do in the bed as you would for Level Two, with bed protection underneath and covering them for dignity.

Digital Decompaction shouldn't ever really be used. But in those rare cases, you are going to be at the beckoning of a finger to help pull out the disgruntled poo. This is not recommended, but if you are going to do it anyway, no one can stop you. Done wrong or too much will result in excessive bleeding. Blood will be present due to trauma and broken blood vessels, which can eventually heal. If you do choose to go this route, at least do it right.

1. Use petroleum jelly and gloves and start around the rim, circling in and around the poo rock
2. Hook into it and pull down and out. If blood shows its face. STOP!

Digital Decompaction is usually something a licensed professional does. So, if need be, see one of these people: RN, LPN, PA, or Physician.

*TIP: Rubbing the lower belly and lower back may soothe the discomfort for your Loved One.

*TIP: Eyeballing the amount of output is good for your documentation for all levels.

Remember to prepare for success by having all cleaning needs available. Whichever process you use can take a while or happen quickly. Like giving birth, you need to be patient.

If none of this works for you, seek medical attention. Medicines are horrible for the digestive tract and the bowels. Messed up, I know, but try to find the lesser of the evils.

If going too much is an issue and they don't feel good, feed them the BRAT diet: Bread, Rice, Applesauce, Toast. BRAT!!!

OMG! Messes

It's all over the place! What to do?!?

Plan your direction of attack that flows easiest for you. You will need a list of things to grab.

Grab List

1. Trash Bin - make sure it is big enough to hold the total mess
2. Dirty Linen Bin - preferably not a decorative one. I don't want you getting your best bin and then get mad if poo is on it.
3. Two Water Basins – one for wash and one for rinse to contain dirty and clean water used.
4. Tons of Disposable Wipes
5. Two Washcloths
6. Disinfectant Wipes or Spray (human safe)
7. Gloves - you might want to double up for a smooth transition.
8. Replacement Linen – whatever is soiled or has poo on it, change. Normally everything changes no matter if poo is visible or not, but if you don't have extra then only change when visibly soiled.

Refresher

1. Gather your Grab List and extra of whatever can possibly be dirty before you start.

2. Prepare for both the expected and the unexpected.

    a. Position everything needed in a way to flow with the task from beginning to end.

Always clean is these directions:

1. Clean to Dirty - makes a big mess smaller than what it can be. If you don't believe me, I dare you to try the opposite way. Wait. No. Never mind. Just trust me on it. I don't want your Loved One to suffer more than they already have to.

2. Front to Back - prevents the chance of infection from poo. After being pushed down and to the back, leave it when you turn over to clean the back side.

3. Wipe down and away - collect all soil in the middle of the pad away from the clean linen and the booty and roll up like a subway sandwich. As you roll it up, pull it away. Then toss it. And finish cleaning and apply the creams and underwear of choice.

Colostomy Care (Poo Bear Bag)

When one has these things, they become insecure. Any stench smelled around, other people will automatically assume it came from them because of this bag. Please do not respond to anything you smell in a negative and judgmental way.

Having this bag means it needs to be Monitored, Cleaned, and Changed.

First let's understand the colostomy part. Colon + Stoma = Colostomy. This is a part of your large intestine or colon connected to the stoma (opening). This means the healthy colon is tied to an opening through the stomach to bypass the rectum. Rarely, though, pooping through the rectum can still be still possible. I have seen some things in my day.

This is their way of going #2 now. Once they have gone, we have to empty the toilet (colostomy bag). Toilets need cleaning and so will these. You can even replace these bags more than you can an actual toilet.

Caring for the Colostomy

Monitored - keep an eye on this bag as it fills through the day - empty or change - from time to time. Release the air out of it also known as burping.

Emptying and Cleaning

Level One

Sitting in a chair and leaning over the toilet is the easiest. They can even stand over the toilet. I have to say, though, that is a high dive for back splash. Don't give yourself a mess when you logically don't need one. Then wipe the inside and outside of the opening until there is no more poo on your toilet paper. Go over outside with a wet one and then close that puppy up.

Level Two

This is for a Loved One that can sit up but is only able to hold a bowl. Sitting up, give your Loved One a bowl with a durable bag lining it (no holes). They should hold it underneath the bag opening, squeeze it empty, and then clean it with dry and wet wipes. Double-check the bag after you close it. Take the durable bag out of the bowl and twist it and tie it closed, trapping the poo.

Level Three

This is lying down on the bed, protected, of course. Placing the durable bag on the bed under the stoma so the colostomy bag can empty into the one you will throw away.

Repeat the cleansing process for both Levels One and Two. The cleaning process is all the same, it is just the positions on how to approach it.

Grab List for Changing A Colostomy Bag

- Bag
- Wipes
- Wound Cleanser or Antiseptic Cleanser
- Trash Bag (durable and with no holes)
- Gloves
- Scissors
- Alcohol Wipe
- Adhesive Wipe
- Stoma Powder
- Adhesive Paste (optional)

1. Wash your hands and put on your gloves before you start touching.

2. On the new colostomy bag, pre-cut the hole in the middle to a little larger than the circumference of the stoma. Not too big. We don't want too much skin exposed. I would follow the cutting guidelines on the bag and find the ring size to cut one notch bigger than the stoma size.

3. While the trash bag is positioned under the stoma to collect what falls, pull up on the edge of the adhesive part stuck to your Loved One.

4. As you peel it off and away, keep the bag upright so the poo inside doesn't fall out.

5. Place the used colostomy bag in the trash bag upright to contain the mess.

6. Clean the visible poo off with wipes, but if it's too dry, you may have to wet it more instead of rough wiping.

7. Rinse off and clean again with wound cleanser dabbing dry after. Tie the trash bag securely and discard.

8. Wipe the skin around the stoma so that all the skin the adhesive will stick to is wiped with alcohol. Let dry.

9. Have wipes ready to grab any poo that might come out of the stoma while cleaning it. You can blame stimulation. Haha.

10. With the powder, slowly and thinly pour a ring around the stoma, trying not to touch it. This can burn after a while and the powder is for the bag purpose.

11. With the adhesive paste, put a ring around the edge of the sticky part of the bag. This will help adhere to the skin with no leaks.

12. Now, make sure the opening at the bottom of the colostomy bag is closed and secured, place it over the stoma and align so the stoma is in the middle of the hole you made bigger.

13. The opening of the bag should be downward and tilted to the side a bit. This will stop the bag from getting in the way when sitting down.

14. Press down and around the stoma so all has adhered.

15. Discard the trash and put everything away. POW!

16. Wash your hands.

*FRUIT: There are always two sides to everything; a story, a coin, and a burp. LOL

Hygiene and Dressing

This section covers everything I can think of, from all types of hygiene, dressing, touching back onto O.T., and getting through the day. Understand this is a time to exercise your knowledge of your Loved One's autonomy and respect that as much as possible, but if it has been too long, they need to get cleaned and I understand. Please don't pass the judgment boundary, considering it is a thin line to cross. Know when it is time to be objective and subjective. To be in someone else's personal space, you must keep your feelings to yourself and take the attention off their naked body.

For the HYGIENE part of this section, we hit a CORE protocol needed to give the best possible care. It's called "**PEACE!**"

Prepare everything first.

Explain what you are doing.

Assist with what they need.

Complete/**C**lean what they can't.

Eliminate as you go by having a laundry and trash bin nearby.

This is what you will follow during any bathing technique. What are the bathing techniques? Well, you have the main understanding behind all, either a **Complete** bath (from behind the ears to between their toes) and **Partial** bathing vital and smelly areas (underarms, breasts, and bottom).

All bathing is much the same, with the result being clean. Let them choose, along with their capabilities. No forcing.

But there are different ways of bathing. For example,

1. Shower (self-explanatory)

2. Tub Bath (sitting in the tub) - a quick tip for this is to have them sit on a towel for friction which also makes it easy to get out. Prepare to get in with them to get them out.

3. Sponge Bath (buckets nearby for bathing or at the sink) - quick tip, keep them covered with towels for dignity and/or if it's cold.

4. Bed Bath (exactly what it is, a bath in the bed) - you don't have to soak the bed; however, you will have to keep towels warm and on them the entire time and possibly change the linen while you are at it.

5. Bird's Bath (aka vitals). I know this one goes by many names. See how many you can think of.

All bathing should include the face and hands.

When ready to bathe or shower, consider the factors against you.

Loved One's reason for refusing.

    a. Bad shower memories
    b. Depressed (let them know they will feel good after)
    c. Dignity
    d. Time of routine
    e. Ill or feeling sick
    f. Feeling rushed through it
    g. Fear of water or drowning
    h. Overwhelmed at the moment
    i. The temperature of the water or baby, it's cold outside
    j. Even bad lighting

That's why you should go over your Safety, Communication, Procedure, and Environment with your Loved One to ease their minds into thinking that you know what you are doing.

Keep in mind an earlier *FRUIT…you will be dealing with one of the three traits we carry within ourselves.

1. The Compliant
2. The Compromiser
3. The Contrary

For the contrary, you need to work a little harder at persuasion. No one is to be forced physically to the point of becoming abused. It will turn into another bad shower memory and they won't trust you in the bathroom ever again.

These traits may determine in what way the bathing process will go. That's why you have so many things to choose from.

Distractions for the child inside would be good, such as a music playlist. Their music, not yours. And keeping them covered as much as possible. It is vital for their dignity and a sense of boundaries.

I'll speak about the easy first and then get to the technical. But first, how are you doing?

You should ask this every chance you get to make sure they are comfortable with what's about to go down next.

Chapter 13: Baths

A complete bath is exactly what it is. A COMPLETE BATH. This is where you reach every nook and cranny of the body. Especially if you can't get them into the shower to let the water rinse off the gunk. This covers from behind the ears down to between the toes. Washed, rinsed, and moisturized.

Baths are a personal thing that most people do in private and we as caregivers only want to be there for support. Having everything they need so they may do it in the order as they see fit. But, if you are the one to delegate or do the work, make sure it is set up to your liking quickly and efficiently. A bath takes longer than a shower normally; therefore, you may need to reheat or change the water during the process. If feasible, always keep your Loved One covered and warm.

What you need:

- Two buckets for washing and rinse
- Two washcloths (third one in case one gets dirty)
- Soap
- Lotion
- Wipes (for unexpected messes and private regions)
- Towels (keep in dryer for warmth)
- Clothes (to dress in what they want to wear)
- Blanket (putting the blanket in the dryer while you finish everything and lastly put it on them to end in warmth)
- Music (it's good to listen to music while you bathe. It makes it a more comfortable environment and more inviting to do it again)
- Water (get the water last so it stays warmer longer)

Every time you wash an area, rinse, dry and cover it back up. Repeat this until all body parts are washed. Lather lotions and cover until you are ready to dress. Remove items no longer needed for they may cause obstacles to continue the process. By the end, they will be ready to dress. Don't leave them exposed or naked. I can't say this enough.

You can bathe in any order, but for me, I do it this way:

1. The Hair
2. The Face
3. The Body
4. Shave
5. Mouth/Teeth

The Hair - Shampooing

*TIP: Cotton in the ears is great for helping to keep the water out though it is inevitable for them to get wet.

There are different ways to shampoo the hair.

- There is a dry shampoo spray for people who don't like to get their hair wet. I don't care for this one. It is like a sanitizer, only good a time or two before you have to wash.
- There is a "no rinse" liquid shampoo and a "no-rinse" shampoo cap. These two can be used a few more times than dry shampoo, but I recommend washing with real rinsing water as they don't always get the whole job done. You can also stick the bottle in a jar of hot water to warm up and the cap in the microwave for fifteen to twenty-five seconds.

- You have regular shampoo and conditioner wash for the shower. You can also have them over the kitchen sink. When putting them over the sink, watch for vertigo and the temperature of the water. Also, having a folded towel to lean on helps.
- You can also wash their hair sitting in a chair with a disposable pad and towel on the floor and another towel over the shoulders, holding a bucket under their head and dousing their hair. Set the bucket down to lather and repeat for a rinse. They're going to get wet, this is a given, so wash the hair first when bathing.
- When they are bedbound, there is an inflatable hair-washing basin for long hair. Keep a bucket nearby for the collection of excess water/drainage. If you don't have it like that, use an inflatable baby bath and prop them up with pillows, for elevation support and head tipping backward (that's what I did for my mom). Shampoo basins are expensive compared to baby baths and they are pretty much the same without the drain.
- The most common way for hospice patients is to put a towel on the bed, under their head and then on top of that, a disposable chuck to catch the excess water. Don't use too much shampoo, you will be forever rinsing and run out of drainage pad. Next, it'll go all over the bed, which you'll have to change. It won't matter if you plan on changing the sheets. That's why you do the hair first. When you are done, tuck in all the pad corners and dispose or it will pour out onto the floor. Boom!

Keep hair brushed so you don't end up with a bird's nest. When brushing/combing hair, start from the bottom and end at the scalp. If you can, section it off so you are not so overwhelmed. For the more tender head, take a section of hair and twist it by the scalp tight enough and hold, you can brush and it does not hurt as much. Spreading the hair helps find possible holes for separation to divide and conquer that nest.

The Face

Here is the face diagram to wash. After each spot in the area, move to a clean part of the washcloth to continue the wash. If the washcloth gets cold, wet it again to make it warm, and then continue.

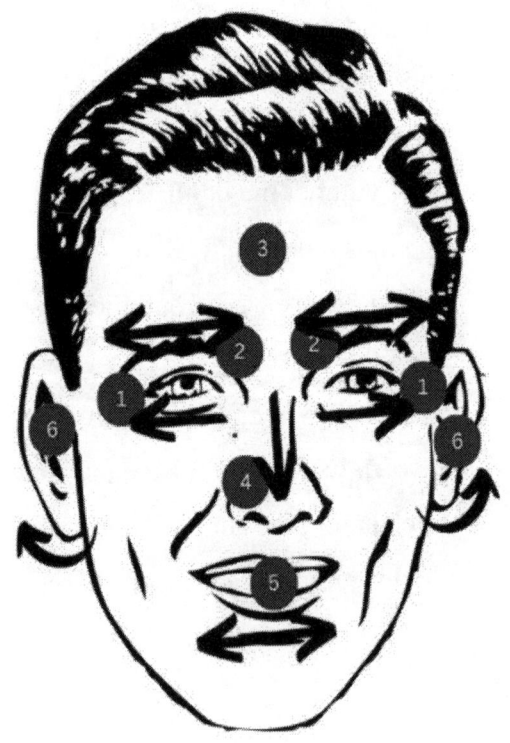

174

1. Eyes – Get in the corners, wiping away, and look for wild eyelashes.

2. Eyebrows – Feels so good, you don't know. Don't forget the unibrow area.

3. Forehead – Don't rub too hard; side to side does the trick.

4. Nose – Down the shaft and the side creases. Don't forget under the nose. Booger city.

5. Mouth – Pay attention to the sides of the mouth and around the lips as this can become crusty and washing this area makes the skin feel revived.

6. Ears – Go with the valley grooves of the ears, pushing everything out before you reach the ear canal. Don't forget behind the ear and lobe.

7. Neck

8. With a beard, wash it like the head with shampoo. My Dad would have specks of food and tell me his beard was his "Flavor Saver."

For the Rest of the Body

1. **Chest** – For women, make a Figure 8 while getting under the breast and wipe everything to the forefront and center. You'll know what they have eaten that day. Don't forget to clean the breast and nipple area. Unfortunately, I have seen my share of booby rocks. Check the navel. You might find one there too.

2. **Pits** – wash what you see and look for what you can't. The underarms can go deep inside above the rib cage. Have them reach for the sky, but prepare to go in like a cave discoverer if they can't.

3. **Arms** – up and downward motion to take any dead skin off.

4.   **Legs** – do the same as you do to the arms. Please get the back of the knees, this is commonly missed.

5.   **Back** - you can wash for them (they may appreciate it). Wash vigorously with a little scrub and wipe off with hand while rinsing with water. For the more sensitive, be gentle, yet thorough.

6.   **Feet** – some people like to wash their feet themselves though if they can't reach, it becomes your job. Scrub all over the feet; on the bottom, heel, under and between the toes and make sure they are rinsed after. Get all that yellow cake off their feet. It's like the yellow cake on the hands, wax like.

7.   **Private Parts** – the region between the upper thigh and the bottom of the navel.

- Standing - if they can stand, great you can see everything better.
- Sitting - have them lean to the side as far as possible, preferably towards a wall, better chance of stability and a better cleansing.

Your Loved One can lean far forward so you can clean the back.

I saved perineal cleaning for last because it is the most extensive. You want to make sure they are properly cleaned and no CHEESE is left behind. It will build upon itself and eat the skin underneath.

What is the cheese you say?

It is the gunk that builds up of dead skin and compilation of creams and any other gunk that, I don't even want to know. We all have it; we just don't let ourselves get enough to notice it. Well, you just might spot it now and you should know how to properly clean it.

Men

1. Douse the area with water and lather soap all over that puppy. Start from the tip and make your way down. Manipulate the skin so you can clean in the folds all over and wipe out any cheese you see. Douse with water and wipe with a clean wipe or washcloth. Rinse two more times than soaping. Never put your washcloth back in the water if it's too dirty or gets poo on it. That's why you have the 3rd washcloth. But I prefer to use disposable wipes for the messy and washcloth on the clean.

Women

1. Do the same, spreading the lips apart and finding all the crevices and cleaning the same way. Leave no cheese behind. From top of front all the way down and to the back, *never* coming back up to the top. You will pull all the dirty back into the vaginal canal causing worse infections.

For both men and women, this may be tender and if hasn't been cleaned properly for quite some time, may hurt. Apply a proper barrier cream for these regions and attend to it regularly until redness and sores are gone. Please keep properly cleaned preferably every day or at least twice a week, thereafter.

Rinse after each section and when the water gets cold, add more hot water. Change water to clean hot water when too dirty.

Shaving

Important Shaving consists of keeping the sharp blade clean while shaving. I never suggest shaving with lotion because it will build in the razor and become dull. This will make you use more strokes than needed and irritate the skin.

When shaving, lather and stimulate the skin well before going against the grain for a smoother shave that lasts longer. Shaving multiple directions will catch all the wild and thick hairs. Stretch the skin to go over wrinkles and please try to refrain from pushing too hard. This is a blade and you will nick them good and they will bleed, what feels like, forever.

Face:

1. Wet face with a hot washcloth.

2. Lather area with shaving cream

3. After wiping your hands, stretch the top of the cheek and shave downward in a zig-zag motion, rinsing the razor after each row is done. Side to side will catch the strays. Wipe the cheek off for a better grip stretching the surface you are shaving.

4. Go with the grain, against the grain, sides of the grain, and one last time against the grain for a smoother feel.

5. For a clean cut, repeat this technique all over the desired area with frequent rinsing of the razor. If you don't rinse between each stride the cut will be harder to do, take longer and dull the blade faster. No cutting corners.

6. Rinse the face off with a hot washcloth getting in all the nooks and crannies of the shaved skin.

7. Aftershave or even a moisturizer can help with dryness.

Arms and Legs:

1. Deodorant needs to be washed off if you use it otherwise it will clog the pores in your armpit, causing blackheads.

2.	Wet and Lather with shaving cream

3.	Going up and down in a zig-zag motion will push some of the hair out of the blade making it easier to rinse out. Going up against the grain and down with the grain helps to clean the blade.

4.	Repeat until all hair is loose and rinse off the body freely.

5.	Rinse frequently between long zig-zag strides.

6.	Go over what was missed.

7.	Rinse off with hot washcloth and moisturize.

Private Parts:

Infections and sores may be the cause of having to shave the genitals and the pubic area. If you should need to do this, this is how.

1.	Wash and Lather

2.	Stretch the area and shave with the grain down and a zig-zag motion across the area making rows down. Rinse the blade frequently.

3.	Keeping the skin stretched, rinse to see what needs to be gone over again, and then do so rinsing an additional time.

4.	For the woman's lips region, stretch the lips flat and shave the stretched area. Move positions of stretched skin to get everywhere desired.

5.	If shaved, it's usually the hood part of the vagina because the hairs hold bacteria and cause major irritation. The same with under the scrotum of a man.

6.	I've only had to shave one crack because the man had a hairy hole and every time he went to the bathroom, it was shower time. If you do that, the only thing I can say differently than what you would already know how to do is watch out for hemorrhoids.

7. Please remember not to push down but only glide across the skin with the slightly firm blade.

Mouthcare

It is important to ensure there is no 'build-up' in the mouth. You need to have them rinse at least once or twice a day. Brushing teeth is sometimes hard, so approach with sensitivity and don't jab with the brush. Two cups (one with water and one to spit in) is helpful should they not be near the sink. Brushing teeth is easier inside the shower.

Dentures are scary because they are expensive so, put a washcloth in the bottom of the sink, and wash them over that. If you drop them, there is less chance of breaking them.

Nail Care

Please make sure nails are clean and trimmed for both of you or it will be a cat fight. An Orange Stick (sharp stick for nails) will get the gunk from under the nails. Those nails need to be trimmed so that they may not scratch themselves, or worse, others.

When it comes to clipping nails, you can clip them yourself being very careful not cutting too far down to injure. If your Loved One is diabetic, I suggest filing them down temporarily and then having a professional clip them to the proper length so as not to cause bleeding.

Soaking nails in a bowl of warm soapy water to loosen any crud that shouldn't be there helps ease the cleaning process of trimming the nails.

Cutting at a slight angle for a better view of the blades will ensure a more precise clipping.

Chapter 14: Showers

I don't think I have to go into further detail about how to wash, I just need you to be prepared for "As You Do." Shower washing ends up with the same result as giving a bath – a clean Loved One.

I use the same washing order as if I were giving a bath:

1. The Hair
2. The Face
3. The Body
4. Shave
5. Mouth/Teeth

Preparation is KEY. Ensuring everything is in order, and prepared with the water temperature hot enough yet not scalding, will make the process easier and will give your Loved One confidence they need in you.

I'll give you the list of everything you need to take a shower.

Go to the store and look for three things:

1. a grab bar with suction cups for them to hold on to
2. a hand-held shower head with cord
3. shower chair

These items can make a world of difference when taking a shower. I mean it. Depending on the texture of the shower walls, suction grab bars can be placed where it is more comfortable for your Loved One to hold on to and feel more stable, hence, giving them more confidence to take a shower.

I would say two bars are good enough, but if they have to maneuver more, definitely don't hesitate to buy more depending on your environment. If your walls are textured and you're unable to use the suction cups, permanent bars may be the best route. If falling is in their regular routine, I suggest having permanent grab bars installed no matter the texture.

A shower chair is a must. I know they are still independent, but what if they get tired of standing and they are still all soapy?

BOOM!

Shower chair! Okay so if a shower chair comes up to be small for your butt or you need more room to get in, I suggest a shower bench. It is a longer seat that has two legs in the tub and two legs out.

*TIP: The curtain will not cover the whole bench chair. However, the chair itself has a crack in the seat that the curtain can fit, lining the shower without getting water on the floor. For protection, I would still put a towel around the two legs outside the tub.

What's that Grampa? You tired? Go ahead and sit, there is a chair behind you.

Love it.

Now during these crucial times, it's the most convenient time to do a skin check. Say what? Yes, a skin check. Keeping tabs on all changes, bumps, and bruises to the skin is vital and should be reported to the nurse for many reasons.

Prevention of additional care needed, abuse, infections, I mean the list goes on. It also helps the professional know if your Loved One is falling and lying about it. Please believe me, they'll lie to you too even if you are their favorite.

Again and again, I say, preparation is key in order to have a fast and efficient shower.

Have the following prepared to act as your shower grab list:

1. Towels
2. Toiletries
3. Clothing
4. Music (optional)
5. Heater
6. Laundry and Trash Bin
7. Water – heated to the right temperature, ready for them when they join the party
8. Hand Towel or Shower Mat - on the floor of the shower or inside the tub (under their feet)

Let them do their routine, only being an extra set of hands and reminding them if/when they forget.

Level One

The Order of Action is:

1. Undress
2. Transfer into shower
3. Wash
4. Rinse
5. Dry
6. Transfer out of shower

7. Apply Creams

8. Dress

So, get ready first by heating the water temp first. They don't want to sit around waiting naked, if they can't make money off of it more times than not, they don't want to do it. Don't forget that it's colder for them than you. You're still clothed. Now, this goes with all baths and showers. Please prepare before they have to wait.

With more mobile people, they will say to you, "I can take a shower by myself." In this situation, this may be true; however, you should still be on stand-by for safety reasons. They don't always get that, let them know. Respect their wishes and do what you can, start the water, check to see if all safety precautions are in place, throw a couple of towels in the dryer and tell them "You are taking a shower by yourself, I'm just waiting in the wings in case you need something." And sit by, vigilant for any circumstance to arise for your hero work.

If you get to sit on the toilet waiting, this doesn't mean get on your phone. Should they stand up while you are distracted and fall, then that's all she wrote. Even sitting down is a disadvantage starting point. Stand in the wings (sides of the curtains) and make sure if needed, you are there, with no delay in time. Another thing that can help put you and your Loved One's mind at ease, is a shower mat or nice-sized hand towel on the floor. When the hand towel is wet, it also helps keep friction.

Level Two

It is similar to Level One, but you are doing at least half, if not all, the work. You can tag team their body by having one washcloth and giving them one as well, washing all over and keeping them warm with the water at all times. Don't be afraid to get wet. It's inevitable and don't be a baby about it.

The Order of Action.

1. Undress
2. Transfer into shower
3. Wash
4. Rinse
5. Dry
6. Apply creams
7. Transfer out of shower
8. Dress

To apply creams is optional in or out of the shower. It all depends on your Loved One's opinion along with yours.

When they stand up on a mat or towel, I still think you need to secure their legs from sliding by holding the shin area to help prevent any slippage. I live by the "stand tall, hands-on wall." This way, they are safe knowing they have structure support and in return, you can reach the areas that are hard to reach.

Now, I promote independence, so if they can reach it, let them wash it. That goes along with the whole dignity issue. If they aren't getting it well, go ahead and scan over those general regions so we don't have any build-up or missed sores and/or bruises. Let them know that you want to double-check and clean, so they won't itch later.

Make sure they hit all key areas.

*TIP: Washing the hair first, let the conditioner sit in the hair while washing the rest of the body. This will soften the hair for easy management. After lathering up and washing the whole body, rinse the hair along with the rest.

When all is said and clean, let them sit back down and cover them with warm towels and let them dry themselves, with your help of course.

After showers you dry the nooks and crannies as well as behind and in the ears.

Level Three

Tricky to shower a bedbound Loved One if you don't have the setup right. You can do everything in the shower, all the way up to brushing their teeth, shaving, and even dressing.

There are 2 Order of Actions for Level Three:

Option One – Prepare for Shower in the Bathroom:

This option is only for when you know how to fully handle your Loved One's safety and want to keep them warm. Closing the bathroom door behind you will trap the heat and depending on whether you undress them right outside the shower or inside will determine when you turn on the water. You wouldn't want to transfer them into the shower fully clothed with water already on because their clothes will get wet.

1. Undress them before transferring into the shower.

2. Alternative Undressing - Transfer into shower fully clothed and then undress. If your Loved One is cold and their bottoms are hard to take off in the shower, undress the bottom half outside the shower before entering, leaving their top on until in the shower. Take their top off right before starting the water to ensure they stay warm as long as possible.

For either 1 or 2 above, give them a towel while waiting for the water to keep them warm.

3. Wash

4. Rinse

5. Dry - Keeping everything dry may be hard. Have an extra towel on hand to dry around your Loved One. Make sure their feet are fully dried in between the toes. People with diabetes acquire sores very easily and should they have one, it is tough to heal, if at all. Skin breaks down easily and is hard to regenerate.

6. Apply creams - Make sure all creams are rubbed in until invisible. No lotion left in between toes, please.

7. Line the shower floor with a dry towel

8. Dress at least the top half of their body in shower

9. Transfer them out of the shower and dress the rest

Option 2 – Prepare for Shower in the Bedroom:

1. Put Loved One on the bed and undress

2. Transfer into wheelchair and position them in front of the shower.

3. Transfer into shower

4. Turn water on

5. Wash

6. Rinse

7. Dry

8. Transfer to wheelchair

9. Transfer to bed

10. Apply creams

11. Dress in bed

This option is the driest way, but has more transfers. It also gives you more elbow room and ensures the safety of your Loved One.

*TIP: Remember, putting the towels in the dryer beforehand will make the after-shower experience nice, pleasant, and toasty.

Chapter 15: Dressing and Undressing

Dressing and undressing are important times to see what kind of reaction clothes will have on your Loved One by seeing if the clothes have any restrictions and physical effects to the body. Anything taken off and put on needs to be readjusted so no twisting of fabric is visible. Don't hide it. Straighten it out. If anything is restricting extremities, it can cause wounds, loss of circulation, and possible further health conditions.

*TIPs: Dress the worst first and undress the worst last, straighten the fabric as you go, loosen before you dress or undress.

TOPS

Level One – Help with how they usually do themselves. Buttons and zippers are not people's favorite so you might be better off dressing them yourself when patience is low.

Level Two – Inserting the worst arm first and then the other. Over or under, but if their arm doesn't move in that way, don't push it. You might want to pick a little looser shirt to put on.

If a pullover, put their arms in first and then let them lift their arms up and pull their head through while pulling the shirt down.

Readjust the sleeves so they aren't twisted.

Level Three – Sitting up would make it best for your Loved One and you; however, if lying down is better for them, you will have a little harder task on your hands.

Dressing the worst arm, pull the rest of the shirt to higher side of their back and tuck it behind the shoulder. Pull the shirt around to the naked arm and have them punch to the ceiling so that you can pull the sleeve on and the shirt down. Lean them forward to do so and then button or zip as needed.

Straighten it down in the back making both sides reach around to the front. Now lay them on their back and button or zip the shirt up.

For a pullover, it's the same strategy; dress the worst arm first, head, then the other arm. Lean forward and pull down, fixing any twist in the shirt and adjust to their liking. The more contracted your Loved One is, the harder it is going to be, so choosing stretchy, loose, and breathable clothing would be best.

Push comes to shove, you may have to cut the shirt up the back. Usually, it is cut straight up the middle while leaving the collar attached. It would look like a homemade hospital gown and guess what. It is! It is open like that for easy access and so you don't get wrinkles behind your back!

BOTTOMS

Level One – Help with how they usually do for themselves and if that doesn't work, assist with how you would do if you were getting dressed.

Level Two – While sitting, dress the legs by putting on underwear, pants, socks, and shoes before standing up. This will limit their energy use and only make them have to stand up once for all clothing items to be pulled up. I also use the "Stand Tall, Hold the Wall" method to complete the dressing. If there is no wall, hold them up by hugging them and use another hand to reach and pull up items. Then let them sit and zip and/or button what's needed. The belt is best put through pants before dressing. Less work for you.

Level Three – This is lying down to get dressed. So, do the same if they sit down and dress the legs first. Pull them up as far as you can get them. If your Loved One is very light, and not fragile, you can hook their legs with your arm going under their knees. lifting their butt, and pulling the pants up with your free hand. Then place them back down gently. If you can't, roll from one side to the next, assuring that all sides are pulled up to the fullest without discomfort. Then zip, button, and buckle.

If they are fragile or heavier than usual, roll them from side to side, continuously pulling up the bottoms and underwear. The better you get at it, the less you roll them from side to side.

If it's men, make sure his package is adjusted to where it's in the front and he is not laying on it and cutting circulation between his legs. A wounded package will be hard to heal if not watched.

SOCKS

Socks SNAG so be careful with these particular items. The threads can also get hung up on the toes and become a tourniquet. Take heed of these. Make sure you change them daily so this won't be an issue**.**

Level One – Assist if needed.

Level Two – There is a device, a sock aid, that can help your Loved One get dressed on their own or help you with great ease. It looks like a piece of PVC that is cut in half lengthwise. The sock will fit over the device on one side while a string will be on the other. Your Loved One's foot will slip into the sock and you can pull the string upwards to have the sock go over the foot. I don't know how much they cost, but you can make one. If you don't have the cutting tools, ask your local home improvement stores if they can help. Then buy the rope and tie it on. A lot cheaper.

Level Three – Place both thumbs in the sock and scrunch it down until the tips of your thumbs are at the toe of the sock. Stretch your thumbs apart, putting the toes in first, guide it over the rest of the foot and pull up.

If you hold the sock to the foot and try to pull the sock on, not meeting the toes together first, a toenail will snag the fabric from the inside and will break a nail or cause another type of wound.

Circulation is problematic at times with socks, so should the socks seem tighter than normal and cause indentations in the skin, slit the top (opposite of where the toes go) with scissors so it doesn't restrict circulation in any way. Just a little slit in the sock can go a long way toward better circulation and comfort.

If it can't fit, don't force it. Cut it. My cousin Becca was doing a puzzle with me and her piece wouldn't fit. She swore up and down it went there. After I put my piece in its place, she said there! She cut it to fit.

Pull a little on the tip of the sock so that the toes are not crammed into the front of the sock. You'll end with a hole like my puzzle.

Compression socks can be worn at any age. I should know, I do. But there is a trick to putting them on. Stabilizing the foot with your knee or leg and with both hands, gather the sock over your two thumbs to the tip of the sock. When all toes are in, carefully pull the sock up, slowly letting out the sock so it evenly distributes up until you reach the top with no wrinkles.

Slightly fold the top part of the sock down so it is smooth and the end doesn't land in the knee crease. Irritation city!

Using the sock aid to dress compression socks is an experience so try your hardest and the more times you do, the easier it gets.

SHOES

For any level, blister protectors can be worn for the blister prone. Keep in mind, the easier the shoe is to take off, the more chance it has of being a hazard. If the shoe doesn't fit, don't make it. They'll be complaining later. And last but not least, shoelaces are tied to their comfort.

Level One – Assist as needed. Offer a shoehorn. I don't care what anybody says, I think Velcro is cool. There are hacks on how to rejuvenate Velcro.

Level Two – Loosening the laces and stretching the tongue so it has a broader mouth for the foot to enter. Don't forget the shoehorn.

Level Three – With loosening the laces and moving the tongue out the way, Turn the shoe slightly and watch the little toes go in at the same time as the big toe will ensure the little toe isn't cramped under the foot. And then, pull the tongue up and tighten the laces from the toes to the ankle. Check the heel and make sure the back of the shoe is out properly and not folded. Again, shoe horn.

Chapter 16: Getting Through the Day (Morn thru Night)

Preparation is KEY. Having each step of your day mapped out is a good start; however, it won't always go as planned, so be a fish and go with the flow. Your days will run into each other, so differentiate the days by doing something special and fun. It's not about existing. It's about living to the fullest of capacity for you both.

Every day will be different and should be taken with day-by-day value. Whether it is a doctor's or salon appointment, make your day around the important tasks at hand.

Ideal List to Follow

This is a list of everything you hope to accomplish for the day. Some days will be a down day and this is where your Loved One can do anything they please. Whether it is going out or staying in and sleeping. Please do not force them to do anything they do not wish to do. Pressuring it too long will turn into force and that is a boundary that breaks trust.

GOOD MORNING

Wakey, Wakey, Eggs and Bakey

It's always good to wake someone up with their favorite beverage while they have time to wake up. In the meantime, for you, this will give you a chance to get everything necessary for your next task.

MEALS

Serve water with all meals and meds as needed. Let them take their time and if you feed them, go slow. Offer sips between bites.

HYGIENE

Whether you do hygiene before breakfast, after breakfast, or before bed, it all coincides with your Loved One's regular routine before you became their caregiver.

This is what your Loved One is doing to be ready for the day. Whether it is taking a shower or a bird bath, they will dress and be prepared. See what times fit best for your Loved One to get cleaned up. Some people like taking showers at night but a good portion like mid-morning. At least once a week. Showering daily causes the skin to dry out faster and lotion is needed more often. Wipe down throughout the week. Please include their hands and face.

For women, a PH balance wash is necessary for private areas.

I prefer liquid over a bar of soap any day. But either way, make sure they are well rinsed off.

Moisturize Daily

DRESSING

Watch the forecast and dress accordingly. If they tend to be colder than usual, dress a little warmer. Dress before standing to complete dressing.

Remember to dress the worst first and the more flexible last. From top to bottom, from hair drying to the shoes.

Remember to stand them up after you have everything on before pulling up the bottoms. One move dressing method.

TOILETING

Do what best fits their bathroom or commode regiment and prepare to check. Wiping from front to back and away. Wet flushable wipes are great and clean better than dry. The dry still leaves a little invisible residue that will leave them itching.

CONTINENCE

Check thoroughly and often to prevent any accidents. Remember to figure out your Loved One's natural bathroom schedule, or as close to as possible, and check before it is too late. Prepare for an accident by having things ready beforehand so they aren't waiting while soiled. Embarrassing for them. Keep that in mind.

AMBULATION

Ambulation is their little way to get what they want or need, watch them, but don't stop them (Level One). If they need help, help them (Level Two). If push comes to shove, go get it for them if it's hard for them (Level Three) and think of it as another way to exercise. If you are helping them walk, remember the walking patterns that fit them better.

BEDTIME

Give medicine an hour or two before bed so that it takes time to kick in. This will also give your Loved One time to wind down from the day's events. This would also be an excellent time to see if they need to go to the bathroom for any reason.

Keep a drink by their bedside for the night. Make sure it's a fresh one that hasn't been sitting there all day.

THROUGHOUT THE NIGHT

Please check in on them. I'm not saying every hour check, just depending on their severity or if they're accident prone.

Helping them to the restroom at least once in the night should suffice.

*TIP: A baby monitor works great for people who may need it. This way you can help them when they need it most and you don't wake them at the most inconvenient times.

Please let them know of the baby monitor if necessary. This will save any awkward moments that might get caught.

When they are stirring on their own, it would be a great time to take them to the toilet and or change them where they stand or lay.

If they cannot move, set the alarm for you to turn and reposition your Loved Ones at least one to two times through the night.

Wake up, rinse and repeat if they feel like it. I promote independence if possible and they want it. Live like no tomorrow and wholeheartedly. Please let them decide what their routine will be each day. The nonnegotiable things are doctor appointments or things considered neglected if left alone long enough.

The following is a reminder of what you need to do for the different levels of Loved Ones. They can sometimes take advantage though, so remember to establish grounds of understanding when enough is enough.

Level One – Make sure your Loved One takes good care of their skin. It wouldn't hurt to look over their body so you may help where they are lacking. This doesn't mean they are moving to Level Two of their care.

Level Two – This is when you have to give your Loved One more attention than usual. You will need to make sure they are done needing your watch before taking it away and on to something else. Leave them in a safe position and all of their needs met.

Level Three – They rely on you "hand and foot." They need to have patience with you and you with them in these harsh times. But understand this is only a moment in time.

Find your routines in how things are wanted to be done. Remember, the end result should be the same and you shouldn't be micro-managed. You both will go crazy and break down.

ACTIVITIES

Give them things to do. They like to do things to pass the time, so throw in some fun things they can experience. Some like to play cards or solitaire. Gambling, you can use pennies or even cheerios, for example.

Some like to dance or go dancing. Keep an eye on them when in motion.

Wisdom to Help You Get Through the Day

*FRUIT: Stop the expectation of others if you can't even have an expectation for yourself.

*FRUIT: If you do not know what to say don't say anything at all as it may be taken wrong.

*FRUIT: There is something about "that person" that I do not like about myself.

*FRUIT: Dear GOD, make my words tender tomorrow, for I may have to eat them.

*FRUIT: Good evening, this is GOD, I will prepare your day for you tomorrow, I will NOT need your help, Have a good night.

*FRUIT: Ask three questions before accepting what is said and before saying what you want.

- Is it true?
- Is it necessary?
- Is it kind?

Chapter 17: Let's Get Out of Here!

When my family and I were ready to take my mom home from the hospital, I told her, "Let's get out of here." In her reply, she yelled, "BYE!" to all the staff and was ready to go.

Because they want to go home, it doesn't mean they want to stay in the house for the rest of their days. Getting out of the house for outings is a moment of feeling normalcy. I want them to get out and I want you to have fun doing that, but for you to have fun, I'm covering a lot of the possible needs while you are out.

To do that:

Preparation is KEY!

Medications

Having all the medicine you need for the day will prevent any issues should you two be out longer than anticipated and therefore have to shorten your outing because of some 'measly' little pills.

Please don't forget a list of medications and dosages taken for your Loved One. Should there be an emergency, the paramedic will know what or what not to give them due to the usage of certain medications.

Sidekick

Let your Sidekick know where you're going. They might want to go and the more the merrier. If something goes down, you have an extra set of hands to maintain the situation.

Jam Bag (for when you are in a jam, of course)

Jam Bag AKA Outing Bag AKA Go to Bag!

Please be prepared for possible accidents and have a couple of clothing changes. One can possibly be all you need, but having a second set will prevent longer embarrassment for your Loved One.

1. Personal Identification Documents and Extra Medication
    a. Driver's License or ID Card
    b. Medication List with dosage and amount
    c. Copy of POA
    d. Medical Insurance Cards
2. Extra Change of Clothes
    a. Tops, Bottoms, and Undergarments
        i. Some disposable underwear and pads (extra protection)
        ii. Suggesting a minimum of four for a 24-hour period. Not including the one they are wearing.
    b. Socks
    c. Sweater or Jacket to keep them warm
3. Extra Cash - a little bit of cash should you run out of items or need a cab ride home if necessary.
4. A Cellphone is a must.
5. Personal Protective Equipment (PPE)
    a. Extra Masks
    b. Sanitizer
    c. Bag of disposable gloves
    d. Tissue and paper towels (a couple)
    e. A couple of plastic bags to discard trash.

Jam Bag is a temporary fix for whatever issues you come across. For some, more than others, a variety of other things may be needed but this is the average. Some people even put snacks in their bag with water or juice (diabetics, etc.).

If your Loved One is medically compromised, and you got it like that, get a portable defibrillator (EAD). When you need it, turn it on, and follow the prompts.

Transportation

Having transportation figured out ahead of time saves a headache on a rainy day. If you don't have transportation, I suggest registering for paratransit in your community. From what I know, you (as their caregiver) or an attendant, can ride as a guest of your registered Loved One. For the most part, you have to arrange transportation two days prior for them. It can be inconvenient as sometimes you will ride around the city before they bring you home. Please remember they are working on accommodating scheduled routes for everyone, not just you guys.

Be Transfer Equipped:

***TIP:** I always suggest bringing a second pair of shoes with more slip resistance and something as simple as a walker with a seat or wheelchair. You can keep it in the trunk of the car if you don't need it right away. Especially helpful if your Loved One can't stand for long periods of time.

What to Expect:

Level One

Will play out like any ordinary day. However, keep an eye on your Loved One and any out-of-the-normal movements and stability issues. If this occurs, treat them as a Level Two for the rest of the day.

Level Two

This is the same as Level One, but I seriously recommend bringing a wheelchair. Walking and adventuring takes a lot of energy and they may poop out before the journey ends.

Level Three

A wheelchair is required because they will be in it all day or until you return home. Keep the venture reasonably flexible should the condition of your Loved One change. As preparation is key, expect the worst and hope for the best when it comes to planning what may happen. I'm not trying to jinx or cause fear, but I just want you to be prepared in case something comes up.

Scenario: what if the condition of my Loved One changes while we're out and cannot wait for the scheduled paratransit pickup time?

Answer: call and cancel pick up and use your cash stash to get an Uber, Lyft, or Taxi that is handicap accessible. If an emergency, call the paramedics and you are prepared with your medication and dosage card to give them.

Now if you don't have a sidekick but need help, this is where outside agencies come in handy. Are you still holding on? Good, you're being good at it.

Outside Agencies and What's to Come:

Life is definitely like a box of chocolates. You don't know which ones you'll get unless you read the picture reference. LOL

In which case, if outside help is needed, you must research which agency is best for you.

If you need extra assistance, then HOME HEALTH AGENCIES are what you need. However, if your Loved One was given a life expectancy, usually 6 months or less, you'll need HOSPICE.

The following chapters will cover what's expected from the outside agencies to last chapter of life and, in most cases, the inevitable ending.

I know this might be a difficult chapter to get through; however, I will try to give you the knowledge as best as I can to prepare you physically, mentally, and emotionally.

Chapter 18: Outside Agencies and What They Do

The main thing you need to know is you are not the only one going through these things and so therefore you are not alone. Outside Agencies are a beneficial service to you so please take advantage of them if available. Research the local services that would pertain to you and then come up with a system with all the services you receive. A lot of the time, services can't be used at the same time. Each service records and documents dates and times with the government, if funded. If you do have two at the same exact time, "Pop" goes a red flag and your help will be snatched out from under you so fast should they think you are using and abusing.

Outside agencies are usually covered by your insurance depending on severity and qualifications. Please be aware that agencies not covered by insurance will need to be paid out of pocket. Agencies that I am referring to are the ones that helps with home health nurse, home health aide, housekeeping and such.

A lot of the time, these professionals take on a case load consisting of anywhere between six people a day to ten on heavy days. This also depends on how much time is allowed for them to attend to your needs.

What they don't do

There are many restrictions and companies have a no-tolerance policy of boundaries prohibited. Please become familiar with the boundaries and limitations.

Nurses are called "Case Managers" on the homecare team and they need to know everything so they can give you everything you need and more. So, please be upfront and honest with them.

Aides are there to help, not to take over. You do for yourself as much as you can; what you can't, they will compensate. Please don't take advantage. They don't overhaul your entire house with scrubbing and cleaning like house cleaners. They do light housekeeping, one to two loads while preparing meals and cleaning the environment your Loved One inhabits, depending on the time frame allowed.

PCA & CNA (There "IS" a Difference)

Personal Care Attendant (PCA) is someone who can help with everything Except:

1. Medications
2. Vitals
3. Wounds

Certified Nurse Assistant (CNA) can help with everything Except:

1. Medications (they work under a registered nurse)
2. Wet and or medicated wound care (the CNAs are only to dress "dry dressing" on wounds).

Questions and Concerns?

I have a question about scheduling. How does that work?

Scheduling a visit for all of your professionals, where they don't get overlap in time, with you would be best. Keep their schedule in mind, as well as yours. Your professionals will be a group of people that juggles not just your needs but others as well. They fight through their day to stay on the best route to meet your requested visit time frame.

Scheduling

Most people think that when you get on a schedule, the agency can accommodate you with whatever at the snap of your finger. WRONG!

You have to help them as much as you want them to help you. I'm sure they can accommodate to a certain degree. Keep in mind, though, that you are only one visit out of their 6-10 visits a day. Be patient and try to keep the communication open so you won't have any hiccups or, if so, they'll be kept to a minimum.

Agencies work better in your controlled environment if you have a structured set-up and schedule, or at least scheduled time frames they know are appropriate for you and your Loved One.

Just like the utility companies, agencies work off a window of arrival, but use communication to generalize a good time agreed. They strive for that time but don't ding them if they are late.

A regular day would be great if it looked like this:

Daily Calendar		
Time	Appointment	Notes
06:00 - 06:45 AM	Visit 1	Wonderful start to the day
06:45 - 07:00 AM	Travel	Travel to next visit - 15 min/mil radius
07:00 - 07:45 AM	Visit 2	
07:45 - 08:00 AM	Break	Have a break, you deserve it!
08:00 - 08:15 AM	Travel	Travel to next visit - 15 min/mil radius
08:15 - 09:00 AM	Visit 3	
09:00 - 09:15 AM	Travel	Travel to next visit - 15 min/mil radius
09:15 - 10:00 AM	Visit 4	
10:00 - 10:15 AM	Lunch	Have lunch Ooh! I love mystery lunches
10:15 - 10:30 AM	Travel	Travel to next visit - 15 min/mil radius
10:30 - 11:15 AM	Visit 5	
11:15 - 11:30 AM	Travel	Travel to next visit - 15 min/mil radius
11:30 - 12:15 AM	Visit 6	
12:15 - 12:30 PM	Break	Have another break!
12:30 - 12:45 PM	Travel	Travel to next visit - 15 min/mil radius
12:45 - 01:30 PM	Visit 7	
01:30 - 01:45 PM	Travel	Travel to next visit - 15 min/mil radius
01:45 - 02:30 PM	Visit 8	
02:30 - 03:00 PM	Head Home	Go home all happy

HAHAHAHA! Did you have your laugh yet?

Here's my rant.

It doesn't look like that in real life. Instead, it looks more like this:

Daily Calendar Time	Appointment	Notes
06:00 - 07:15 AM	Visit 1	Late arrival because didn't put gas in the car the day before
07:15 - 08:00 AM	Travel	Traffic jam and 20 miles away
08:00 - 08:30 AM	Visit 2	Persuade shower and still refuses
08:30 - 09:00 AM	Travel	Travel to meet other C N A - shared 15 miles
09:00 - 09:30 AM	Waiting	Waiting for C.N.A. to arrive who is also delayed
09:30 - 11:00 AM	Visit 3	Have to explain things because you're not the regular CNA that they're used to. Visit 3 still doesn't know why there has to be two of us which then makes us explain further to ease the patient's nerves-delaying us longer.
11:05 - 11:10 AM	Almost Lunch	Pulling into a drive-thru for lunch and the phone rings. It's the office. Someone has soiled themselves and the wife can't turn him. Now they lay in their own mess and need help ASAP!
11:10 - 11:30 AM	Travel	Travel - Lunch should stay cool in shaded parking and by the arrival time it should still be crisp. NOPE, NOT TODAY!
11:30 - 01:30 PM	Visit 4	Visit 4 happened to have passed right before you got there. Not only do we do postmortem care, the RN gets another call after pronouncing and then looks back and says, "I have to go. Stay with them until they are comfortable alone or until the funeral van arrives?"
01:30 - 02:00 PM	Stay	We check their comfort levels before leaving. If they're not in a good space then we stay.
02:00 - 03:00 PM	Lunch	Finally, get back to the car and then realize, lunch was waiting. The fresh cold sandwich turned hot and the bread is soggy yet hard on the ends. Well, on to the next...

I could go on, but you catch my drift.

By the time all patients are done, you get to go home from a hot day in the sun or cold winter slick roads. Let's not talk about the traffic; other motorists shouldn't be driving! Now if one of these people describes you, please don't take it as a complaint. I'm just trying to paint a picture of how a regular day goes for the outside agency that comes out to help. If the motorist sounds like you, I can't help you there. That was a complaint.

This would be different in a more controlled environment between patients (like a group home or facility), but not everybody lives next door to each other. If they have a scheduled time frame and they stay longer than an hour, you're lucky because usually, they have up to an hour unless an emergency. Other possibility is the company has certain allotted hours per week, per overall hours in a year, that's covered by insurance.

Now the Agency should respect the times set and communicate when running outside the lines of that. Flexibility on both parties is what makes this little world of ours go round. Granted, it might be a tight rope, flexibility and all, but anything is better than nothing, don't you agree?

*FRUIT: Just remember to give the same courtesy because what you give out is nine times out of ten what you get back.

Now, I know there are professionals out there that rub you the wrong way on the first visit. I only ask that you give them the benefit of the doubt and let them come one more visit before you decide that they aren't a good fit.

Should they come out the second time and you definitely know the chemistry is NOT there between the two of you, then it is ok to request another professional closest in the zoning area. Just remember a professional that comes to cover your regular aide is sometimes pulled from their zone and may need more time to get to you. So please be patient.

Please speak with all the professionals available to you because each one governs different things you need and keeps you in the loop. If it's something important, please don't be afraid to send the message through multiple staff members. Do not rely on addressing an issue that's important to you only once and please don't think you're going behind someone's back by addressing something important to you to multiple people. Once again, you are the captain of this ship and should be running a tight one. Know all the who, what, when, where and why, I don't care about the how, it better get done!!!!!! I feel like a boss right now saying that.

Sorry about that. Back to the message at hand.

Chapter 19: Hospice

What is Hospice Really?

When someone is imminent has a life expectancy, Hospice is what you want on your side. This service has the main goal of quality care and comfort for your Loved One. It's what they strive for.

Though all Services' main goal should be quality, Hospice has quality along with comfort which is needed most in the final hours. They don't lack in the quality department. It takes a certain special somebody to do that type of job.

Whether we would like to admit it or not, we're all going to die one day and if our passing isn't instant, there will be a moment when you feel like you are running out of time and trying to prolong it. In most cases, it takes longer than you think. In some cases, it hits you like a truck from nowhere. I highly recommend ALL people make their final arrangements ASAP. I don't care if you're sick or not. Death can come whether you are ready or aren't. But when you realize it's not how LONG you have left and it's really about WHAT you do with the time you DO HAVE, life will be more filling on both ends of the spectrum.

Understand that when people hear the word **"Hospice"** and are given a life expectancy, this is a professional's educated guess. It is exactly what it is, an **Educated GUESS** and they **don't know exactly when you will die**. They are saying if this path keeps going this way, they see the evident. What I noticed is when you tell people they are going to die, that is when they, in fact, start to die. They give up. However, fighters out there will go kicking and screaming, last longer than expected and even defy the odds.

What is Hospice Service?

Hospice is a 24-hour, seven days a week, supporting service for you and your Loved One during a terminal illness. It has been reported that people have progressed in good health and were able to "graduate" from this service. And I was not informed of the time after, how long anyone has lasted, but I have seen people get better. Graduated only means that they no longer meet the requirements to qualify for hospice and or show a life expectancy longer than six months. This can always be appealed should you feel they need more time on service.

How to Know if You Qualify

When a Physician suggests that Hospice is the only other option besides fighting with treatment and writes a referral, it won't sink in until you get that paper that says hospice.

To help with these programs, going to the doctor and having a referral is necessary to make the process go smoothly. But to get the go-ahead, they need to know if there is a failure to thrive and some ways to do so are:

1. Voluntary lack of or refusal of nutritional value
2. Unexplainable and continuous muscle/weight loss
3. Terminal medical conditions with a life expectancy of six months or less

The list is revised periodically, so I suggest personally looking into that matter when it doesn't meet the above criteria.

What To Expect

When signed onto hospice care, an "assessment" will take place seeing all that you need and would benefit from what is offered. You'll be assigned to a group of professionals zoned in your area, which include but are not limited to:

1. **Dr., PA and NP**
    a. Physician, Physician's Assistant and Nurse Practitioner are the ones who sign off on the orders requested by the RN and are the deciding factor in care plan.
    b. They should come out on average once a month or two.
    c. It's usually for recertification and or upon request.

2. **RN Case Manager**
    a. A RN who is assigned to govern your care.
    b. These people are the ones that manage your medications, care plans, doctor's orders, wound care, aide schedules and any special needs.
    c. Typically is ordered once a week unless more visits are needed due to the severity of your Loved One.

3. **Social Worker**
    a. When you need help with other things like financial matters, other services or resources.
    b. Pretty much you got a question and need help. They are the ones to go to. No question is a stupid one. Only stupid answers.

4. **Chaplain**
    a. Spiritual guidance and emotional peace are what these people are experts on.

  b. I understand many people don't want to see a chaplain, which means this is really happening.

  c. You need to give them a chance. They are much more understanding than you think and no judgment occurs in their presence.

  d. They have helped me in my most time of need and I am elated that they were available for my emotional well-being.

5. **Aide**

  a. AKA your best friend. Just kidding.

  b. But these people are the ones you will see the most.

  c. They are Certified Nurse Assistants who assist the Nurse and do the grunt work. DOO-DOO! They are the ones that will be giving you a break with strenuous care.

  d. Mainly bath, showers, feeding and wound care assistance (if needed, dry dressing only). Please remember, they do NOT help with medications. Call your RN Case Manager.

  With each of these professionals, please inquire about their profession and what will benefit the situation. They are able to educate you more of what to do in their absence. As far as what you need, they can provide these things. Please inquire of what you need help with accomplishing. Make a list.

Hospice Expectations for Your Loved One's Comfort

1. Safe Breathing

2. Safe Sleeping

3. Safe Eating

4. Safe Toileting

5. Safe Cleansing

6. Safe Ambulating

7. Safe Interaction - Social engagement to their liking. I've seen both party animals and true hermits. Offer bonding time, but if they don't want to, DON'T be overbearing. Find what works.

Medical Equipment

Hospice will provide medical equipment directly related to the comfort and care of your Loved One. Please don't think you won't need any of these things, better to have them. FACT!

What's Given and/or Asked For:

1. Hospital Bed

2. Bedside Table

3. Bedside Commode

4. O2 Concentrator with a Humidifier and Canula

5. Nebulizer Machine

6. Suction Machine

7. Shower Chair

8. Wheelchair

9. Hoyer Lift

10. Trapeze

Please be sure to request portable devices if needed, such as oxygen tanks (along with the holder) or walking devices.

When in doubt, speak to SOMEONE!!! Not ALL of these are a MUST for your Loved One, but these are available should they benefit from it. The first four on this list are the most common and should be standard.

Additional HELP to ask about.

If available, PLEASE ask for all services provided that relate to your circumstances needing resolution. Examples include:

1. **Podiatrist**
    a. May or may not be contracted with the agency.
    b. Speak with a Professional about your options.

2. **Transportation**
    a. May or may not be contracted with the agency.
    b. Speak with a professional about your options.

3. **Pet Needs**
    a. Rehoming, fostering, and other services. Speak about your options.

4. **Groceries**
    a. See about your options.

5. **Therapies** (all types that they provide)
    a. Occupational
        i. Therapy on how to do daily activities for oneself. Dressing, feeding and living.
        ii. This has to be ordered by a nurse through a physician. Strong-Will must be present, which will work their limitations and help them understand

how far they need to go to become completely independent again.

b. Physical
   i. Therapy helps build resistance, muscles and stamina along with flexibility.
   ii. This also has to be ordered by a nurse through a physician and is also restricted depending on level of conditions your Loved One is dealing with.

c. Massage
   i. Stimulates and relaxes tense muscles and contracted limbs, as well as relieves some pain.

d. Reiki
   i. For spiritual touch that soothes peoples' spirits and energy. I'm not too knowledgeable about this, but it is available.

e. Music and Art
   i. I know a few people who took advantage of this for children and the patient and it helps with the process of losing a parent or even going through the dying process.
   ii. Yes, this is also available for your Loved One's suffering, including you.

6. **Volunteer**
    a. A lot of places, if not most, offer Volunteers who are a blessing from heaven when you've got people to see and things to do.
    b. DON'T take advantage. These people are not getting paid but are helping out through the kindness of their hearts. So be considerate.
    c. When YOU have a doctor's appointment, please let the agency know as soon as possible so you can secure that time.
        i. It's kind of like a first come, first serve appointment setting and if they are low staffed that day, you already got your ticket in.
    d. People are volunteering their time and companionship and are restricted on level of help or assistance for your Loved One.
    e. They cannot give medicine and cannot move your Loved One.

7. **Respite**
    a. A temporary five-day or less stay at a Hospice or independently contracted facility. If more than 5 days or at an independent facility, there may be out of pocket expenses.
    b. This is allotted every sixty days; if needed sooner, there must be a valid reason for placement excluding burnout.
    c. Respite is given when

      i. Emergency placement is needed such as a power outage or flooding occurs

      ii. Medical conditions or pain management need to be addressed

      iii. Caregiver burnout affects you and your Loved One.

Please note that when assigned to Hospice, you are NOT obligated to stay with them should you be unsatisfied in any way. It's all about your comfort; if you are unhappy, they are not doing their job to your standards and maybe there is another hospice agency that can comply with all your needs. Ensure you notify the agency of your needs or they cannot give your Loved One the best care. Let the appropriate professional know. They are here for you, not their health, you heard?!

Refresher - Being gentle in these moments of your Loved One's last chapter is crucial and give everything wanted with pure love as if it will be the last, every time.

When your Loved One is in hospice, I want you to implement the HUMAN CHECKLIST. These people are in the last of their days and don't deserve to suffer anymore.

This brings us to the last few pages of their "Life Book."

The care you give your Loved One during these fragile times is slightly different and contradicts what I taught you earlier. They are sleeping more, weak, not eating, and barely or, if at all responsive. It is finally down to the wire and now it is a waiting game. This is when SHIT gets REAL. Care for them until the very last breath. But the things you will do differently will be more explained by WHY you are doing it. If signs of suffering are obvious, comfort meds will help them through anxiety and pain. This medicine is for comfort and not a reviver. Don't think that this medicine they take sends them home or makes them better. Instead, understand that the doses given are only for comfort measures and are there to help with a peaceful passing. Medication is usually refused until unbearable to cope. Some just sleep away. Still, care until the last breath.

Importance to maintain or know why this function occurs.

The closer we get to our end, the more pain and frustration we'll have and lesser control of the body. The functionality of the brain detaches little by little from our bodies. First goes physical control, then consciousness (want to sleep all the time), then nerves, if they haven't already. Our time can be at any time, but for the gradual aspect, it's described like this:

Transitioning - Failure of the Body to Thrive Before Passing

1. Refusal of Everything

At times, we start refusing everything because the body feels it will take too much energy and all we want to do is sleep. At this point, let them do what they want.

2. Unexplained Muscle and Weight Loss

The body will start to shut down because the parts needed to take in nutrition are broken.

For instance, one of the fifteen causes my mother succumbed to, was metabolic encephalopathy. The organs shut down due to the brain not allowing her to take in the nutrients needed for her to heal.

3. Doesn't Want to Eat or Drink

As our organs are shutting down, it sends signals to the brain to stop the hunger and thirst switch. Should people try to eat, the stomach has powered down and the undigested food will sit in the body. A lot of the time, people start to taste chemicals or what seem like metals.

4. Mouth breathing

Mouth breathing is what we resort to when weak and the jaw is too heavy to hold up. The nose may be plugged. If they are mouth breathing, the nose cannula won't get used properly. Taking the nose cannula and putting it over and across the mouth may work until they take it off. Because a good portion of people become mouth breathers, it will feel like a dry desert inside and that's why they'll want water to moisten.

5. **Thirst**

Our body is made up of 60% water and the organs use roughly 75% of that. As we deplete it by sweating and peeing, we try to replenish by drinking more water. At this stage, sometimes moistening the mouth is all your Loved One needs. It's almost as if it's our body's last-ditch effort to prolong the inevitable and we never deny them water, ok?

*TIP: Always offer water every chance you can, though, some people are restricted water and moistening the mouth will help with their feeling of thirst.

6. **Thrush**

It is possible people don't want to eat or drink because it hurts and nothing tastes good due to a white coating you may see in their mouth. If they have this, it may be thrush. This type of fungal yeast infection can only be treated with medicine, mouth wash and oral care. Thrush is painful and leaves redness and sores. It kind of looks like cheese buildup in the mouth. Tell the doctor immediately if your Loved One is dealing with this.

7. **Broken Thermostat**

Hypothalamus is the body's thermostat in the brain and when it breaks it usually causes us to either feel cold to the touch but burning up inside or hot to the touch but feeling chilly. Having a type of cover nearby, heavy or light, to their liking is great. If we cover them up, only for them to continually take it off, let them be. This is their physical way of telling you they are not cold.

8. **Terminal Agitation**

The uneased feeling one gets when one can't get comfortable or situated the way one wants. It will be hard for you because you can't make them comfortable. Go through the problem reliever checklist to do all you can. After that, you may have to resort to medicine for agitation. A little prayer goes a long way.

9. Change in Urine Like Tea or Coffee

This usually means the kidneys are shutting down and proteins (what we have left) are coming out through our urine. This can also explain muscle and weight loss.

10. Wounds

Our bodies cannot heal anymore, let alone stay together. Blood restrictions through the skin cause wounds, inevitably, but can possibly be prolonged for a long while. It will feel like you are losing control of the situation down to the. But you're not. It is the process. You were never really in full control anyway. You only help their transition go smoother. This is where a lot of understanding, accepting, and forgiving should occur before the end.

Actively Dying

This means we have lost our consciousness and can go anytime from now until we pass. When someone can last three weeks without food, three to five days without water, and three to five minutes without oxygen, these can give an estimated length of time left. Before this happens, they will go through some signs before their demise.

Signs and Symptoms

In hospice, they give you a book to explain the signs and symptoms that come with the end stages of life. I suggest you read that and I mean read it. They have mapped out how it would be, but people can skip certain stages and even jump back and forth between them.

Rallying is when they get the last burst of energy and want to do so much, but it ends up exerting them and pushes them closer to the end. In many cases, this can happen a few times but usually once. Don't be surprised if they do it twice.

For the people who still have their hearing, it will be the last of the senses to go so watch what you say. Or say what you need to. They will hear you.

Periodic Tasks to Help

1. Repositioning for Comfort

The more pillows, the better. Give them a bed of pillows so they can sleep on a cloud. The turning to the side needs to be done softly and slightly. Do NOT keep them on their full side. The worry about turning on the side is the weight pushing on the organs. The more you move them, the more stress on the body and the more stress on the heart to pump harder and faster. The body's weight needs to be distributed properly (spread to be lighter) so the weight sitting on the organs won't stress it and speed up the dying process.

Playing music in the background is low enough for them to hear but not so loud it causes them to be irritated. Some people don't really want music and you ask if they can still answer. Soft lighting is appreciated, if any at all. I think many enjoy the company of their Loved Ones. The laughter about memories can put your Loved One there again and they smile, feeling joy. Showing them, they are not alone. But many wait until they are alone to leave and pass away.

There will be a time when you come in and find them unresponsive and with no pulse; Don't panic! You need to be in charge. If your Loved One is a full code, meaning resuscitate, call 911, put on speaker and start CPR.

If they have a DNR (DO NOT RESUSCITATE), it should be posted by the bed on the wall and visible. Set a timer for five minutes for count of any breaths slipping by. If none, please call your hospice or 911. Please let them know if they were a DNR and they will be discreet.

Before you do, you can have a moment with your Loved One that just passed. Please do not wait long because we are biodegradable. And our decomposition will start soon.

2. Oral Care

This is where dent-tips come into play a lot more. These sponge squares on sticks look like fake popsicles and are in place of the abrasive toothbrush.

Using a glass containing 1/3 mouthwash and 2/3 water is good for use up to three days. Leaving the glass container covered when not in use is vital to keeping it fresh longer. When using the dent-tip, dip in and dab it on a folded paper-towel for excess and gently swab the inside of the mouth all the ways possible. Start with the inside of the cheeks all around and if it's not visibly soiled you can return it to the water. I never return to the water if visibly soiled, it'll taint the water and you have to start all over with clean water. If soiled, use another. Every time you clean their mouth, consider that you may use two to three, depending on how dirty.

Be aware that they may bite down when you pass through to the inside of the teeth where the tongue is. Don't pull it out, you can hurt them and worse, they rip the sponge and try to eat it. Just be patient and wait until they let up and take out the dent tip when you see an opening. If they bite down again, be patient and try to wait again. Eventually, they will let up.

Swirling the stick while on the gums and teeth will catch as much saliva and gunk as possible. Visibly soiled, change it.

*TIP: If you run out of dent-tips, use a wet paper towel around your finger or a toothbrush. It'll work just the same. Warning: Don't go into the teeth if you use your finger. You won't come back with it. Our bites are harder than you know with or without teeth.

Chapter 20: When It's All Over

What is left to feel? There is nothing left to feel when you lose a Loved One. Sometimes I feel weightless and suspended in time, with the crushing ache of something ripped from the seams of my heart and where now is a gaping hole of dense disbelief on how this has happened. I truly cannot tell you how to feel. I mistakenly told someone what I truly believed and that it would be okay. I understand where I came from when I said it and now, to be on the other side, these words in this order don't settle well with others. They are still suspended in times of disbelief or utter grief.

It is okay to cry. These are all the emotions our passed Loved One has given us. We are not crying for them but more for ourselves. We miss them so much. Here no more. Remember, crying cleanses the soul; when you cry for someone, you are calling to them and they will come to your heart. Please know they feel no pain, as pain is an emotion of the body.

When your Loved One breathes no more, you still are. Show them what you do for them by breathing for yourself. They want you to live on, become the greatest YOU and make them PROUD.

A lot of the time, understanding the loss leaves no words anyone can say to make you feel slightly better, given the circumstances at hand. The best thing is giving your silence for the loss of your Loved One.

Fast or Slow Death and the Lesser of the Two Evils

One is no less than the other, the only difference is it happening too fast and watching what happened. Knowing why or not knowing why. I couldn't tell you which is worse. It doesn't matter anyway. That's not how people want to be remembered. One wanting to know why it came too fast and the other bittersweet of having them there but suffering all the way.

Just know in the end, we go to sleep eventually and pass. Slowly or abruptly.

What to do then?

After You Think Your Loved One Has Passed

What people don't talk about...

When someone passes, time is needed for family and close ones to mourn if they want to come say goodbye, either before or after they pass (Hospice Term: Expire).

Regardless if your Loved One is in hospice or not, if they are full code (resuscitation needed), and have stopped breathing, please call 911 and perform CPR until the professionals take over. If you do have hospice and your Loved One has a DNR, contact the hospice and not 911 as the hospice will make the arrangements for you.

With Hospice

If your Loved One stopped breathing, time them for five minutes and then decide if the family would like to see them and make the call to the hospice if they have a DNR.

Usually, hospice will come out to pronounce the time of death. They are looking for a pulse and sometimes they stop breathing but will still have a pulse. They will time one full minute with no pulse and will call the time of death and this will be what is recorded on the death certificate. This may differ from what you remember as the last time they stopped breathing.

This is then when you tell the nurse what mortuary you will be using and they will call to arrange for them to be picked up. Please feel free to discuss final arrangements with the hospice prior to their passing which will help with the process.

While waiting for the mortuary to arrive, you can prepare their last and final bath, just as great as the first one. Dress and prepare them for the morgue to pick up. When dressing, if rigor mortis has begun to set in, dress the stiff-side first. You can always alter the clothing to fit properly with a slit here or there.

*TIP: If your Loved One has a DNR and has stopped breathing, it is ok to take your time before calling hospice if you or your family requests extra time with your Loved One's body. But I suggest doing it in a timely fashion, considering nature will take its course and we all know what happens after.

Without Hospice

If you do not have hospice and your Loved One has stopped breathing, please call 911 and let them know. Let them be aware if this is a Full Code (resuscitation needed) or if they have a Do Not Resuscitate (DNR) form. If your Loved One is Full Code, you will need to perform CPR until the professionals arrive. They will then take over and direct what should be done next. Most likely you will need to contact or arrange pickup with a mortuary in your location after the coroner or professional has called the time of death as natural passing.

As hard as it may be to do so, please refrain from touching or washing your Loved One until after the professionals have finished what they need to do.

Understanding

I'm so sorry you have to go through this. I tried to put it gently due to this sensitive matter. Again, I'm sorry.

They say, "You know you are getting older when everyone around you is dying." As we get older, our minds can find the funny side of life with the morbid view of the inevitable. It's being at peace and accepting what is unavoidable. No one can live forever physically.

I didn't understand the full meaning of dying until I heard the words "Here No More." When I heard these words, it touched my soul.

I once knew a terminal young woman who laughed at life, showing no care for dying like it was no big deal. We had a conversation about dying and I had asked her if she was scared. She asked me, "scared of what?" My response was "here no more." I have never been hugged so tightly while shaking and crying with distraught. She kept everyone at bay by playing it off, but none of them were able to understand the full vulnerability because most don't like to be confronted with the idea of death. It makes them think of their own demise and some, more than others, do not want that kind of a reality check. She had not cried the whole time of her illness. She needed to be raw with herself and know she was not alone through this difficult time. Her journey was just beginning and she was no longer a comedian of the times in her eyes, but the love of many.

I just want you to know that you are energy that lives on and transcends you into pure love.

The grieving process starts when given a Life Expectancy.

Time heals what reason cannot.

Coping is something I still struggle to deal with, so suggesting you to "release" it by talking to someone is worth a shot. Stranger, family, friend, professional someone.

Healing – Healing takes time and one day at a time. We will never fully heal until acceptance starts. Take the right steps to help you heal by putting yourself out there and living the most out of life.

Let your Loved One who passed live vicariously through you.

Family – Your family went through it with you, whether you want to realize it or not. They can be a supportive leg to stand on if the dysfunctionality does not override your love for each other. If this is difficult for you, seek professional help and understand it is okay to ask.

Breaking down can be a vicious cycle always resulting in you still needing time. But remember the good memories you had because they are the only things that mean anything great.

Push comes to shove, write everything that you couldn't get over and burn it. Because in this sense, it will be "here no more." Please let go of all anger you hold in your heart and mind because it will make the choice of where you go after here. I guarantee your Loved One has no worries on the other side. GOD makes them leave it at the gate upon entering.

That was my mother's lesson. Learning to forgive others and herself. She waited for the end to be near before she did it, but at least she came to peace with that before she passed.

Life Says "Thank You"

We are reaching the last section of our journey through this book and I want to leave you with what matters most to me in helping you through all your endeavors. Please go over the book again and highlight what means most to you as well. There is also a recap of the FRUIT and TIPS before I speak to the inspiring professional grunt workers, hopefully to uphold the "Promise."

FRUIT for Thought

Here is a compilation of FRUIT of knowledge I took from my own and other people's experiences and all of life's glories.

- Accept what is, practice what you preach, and evolve with experience. This is the key to a happy existence.

- The core ingredient of bedside manner is "having an interest in others without personal benefit."

- All lessons you go through may be the same. However, one degree of difference between them makes a different lesson altogether.

- Remember, time heals what reason cannot. Your mind needs a reason and your heart needs time.

- Love is good; if you work through love a peaceful journey will surely be your path.

- Whether you think you can or you can't, you're right. Your confidence is only as strong as your will.

- When it's done it's done, no turning back. So, calculate the risk and please be at peace with the outcome. Good luck.

- Have sympathy for others for you may be there one day, then we'd be talking about empathy.

- It's not what you have. It is what you feel when you enjoy what you have. HAPPINESS also equals JOY. But understand happiness comes when you find joy in your life. The little joys add up to happiness.

- Control of our minds is what we hold dear, so don't hold it against others if they lose it.

- Making haste makes waste.

- If in doubt, double up while gloving up.

- Sanitizer is not SOAP! You can use sanitizer three uses max before you need to wash your hands.

- Step back from the box to think outside of it, it gives you fresher eyes.

- One's level of care may change, but your Loved One's dignity never lessens.

- The three traits of you: the Compliant, the Compromiser, and the Contrary. Which one will you be today? Keep in mind Murphy's law.

- Nothing is always as it seems. Some people may know how to walk, but not how to eat, speak, or just do…or in any combination thereof. Looks can be deceiving and we remember about ASSUME? Don't assume just because we can do it, your Loved One can as well.

- Please keep in mind, unless these people wear hearing devices, just because they are older or disabled in some way doesn't make them deaf. Stop yelling in their ears! You people know who you are. If that is your normal voice, ok. For others, there's no excuse.

- Stop the expectation of others if you can't even have an expectation for yourself.

- Be patient my friend while the times occur.

- If you don't want to read the instructions, fine don't. But you better read the "Do Not." It is necessary and important. A hard head makes a soft bottom.

- You don't know how appreciated it is until you are the one doing the appreciating.

- There are always two sides to everything; a story, a coin, and a burp. LOL

- If you do not know what to say don't say anything at all as it may be taken wrong.

- There is something about "that person" that I do not like about myself.

- Dear GOD, make my words tender tomorrow, for I may have to eat them.

- Good evening, this is GOD, I will prepare your day for you tomorrow, I will NOT need your help, Have a good night.

- Ask three questions before accepting what is said and before saying what you want.
    - Is it true?
    - Is it necessary?
    - Is it kind?

- Just remember to give the same courtesy because what you give out is nine times out of ten what you get back.

TIPS to Remember

Here is a compilation of tips that you'll find throughout the book:

LOCC Tips:

- Eat when they eat and make sure you prepare an actual meal for yourself. Don't just finish what they left behind. Remember, if you don't care for yourself, there won't be anyone to care for your Loved One. You both will be up sheet's creek without a paddle.
- If your Loved One has to go the hospital, please leave glasses, hearing aids, dentures, and/or any other prized possessions at home, depending on their length of stay as these things are the most commonly lost or misplaced. If they must go with your Loved One, ensure they're kept in a safe space.

Medication Tips:

- When opening a powdered capsule, put a paper of some sort to catch whatever you spill under your medicine.

Medical Equipment Tips:

- With the heat escaping, a concentrator keeps a room warm for the "cold-blooded."
- Colostomy Bags need to be burped. I know, crazy analogy, right? Burped like a baby, releasing the air from the bag. If you don't, they will pop like the stink bomb my brother put in the Christmas tree during the opening of presents.

Repositioning Tips:

- Keeping the four ends of the draw sheet facing downwards towards the feet, will also keep the wrinkles down behind them.

In the Bed Tips:

- Please, be mindful of their back, shoulder blades, and hips. This is usually where more pressure on the body occurs. Reminder, again, that it's very important to rotate them from supine to left, right, or prone. Not a lot of people are able to be in the prone position for many reasons.
- Please do NOT leave your Loved One sitting unattended at the edge. Make sure if left alone, they are secured in their surroundings.
- Before doing ANYTHING with your Loved One, please keep in the forefront of your mind any object that may be attached to their body, such as a Foley bag, IV, etc. Foley bags tend to hang off something. Just make sure you detach it and keep it near your Loved One. I hang it on the back of the belt so it won't be forgotten.
- If you have one side of the bed by the wall and the bed has a railing, put a spacer between the legs of the bed and the wall. This keeps your Loved One from smashing their fingers.

Transfer Tips:

- If your Loved One's Level One cognitive malfunction lasts for more than three days, you might need to consider this the new normal if everything else comes out fine. They may snap out of it. Hope for the good, you know. If they don't, make that doctor's appointment.
- Counting to three while rocking will give momentum to stand on three.
- A slide board is used like a conveyer belt.
- Check, Check, and Recheck. Being absolutely positive is key.

Ambulation Tips:

- Always support their weaker side for ambulation and keep an eye on them leaning to one side more than the other.
- Keeping their feet up on foot pedals will ensure you don't wheel over their feet and legs and they don't fall or slide out. It is also considered a brace point for your Loved One and a sense of control for them to hold their body in the chair if no safety restraint is available.

Changing Tips:

- I know you may not be able to change a brief right the first time, but you will have plenty of time to practice for perfection. Oh yeah! Don't forget to ensure the brief end (with tabs) is on their backside, not frontside, nor too far up their back. You have less in the front to tab on.

To the Toilet Tips:

- After your Loved One has used the toilet and they are ready to stand, put a temporary disposable paper towel of some sort between their legs, covering the new pull-up underneath. This will prevent any after-leakage or additional accident resulting in changing the pull-up again. Been there, done that, bought the T-Shirt and scrapbooked it.
- Now, don't get short with them if they can't stand and dress. People sometimes need to focus more on the task and less on stability so their equilibrium sometimes goes off-kilter. This is where you hold their stability for them.
- Feeling the stability in your poised posture and strong like a cement pillar gives them confidence in your decisions and they will follow your lead. No spaghetti arms.

Enema Tips:

- Rubbing the lower belly and lower back may soothe the discomfort for your Loved One.
- Eyeballing the amount of output is good for your documentation for all levels.

Bathing & Showering Tips:

- Cotton in the ears is great for helping to keep the water out though it is inevitable for them to get wet.
- The curtain will not cover the whole bench chair. However, the chair itself has a crack in the seat that the curtain can fit, lining

the shower without getting water on the floor. For protection, I would still put a towel around the two legs outside the tub.
- Washing the hair first, let the conditioner sit in the hair while washing the rest of the body. This will soften the hair for easy management. After lathering up and washing the whole body, rinse the hair along with the rest.
- Remember, putting the towels in the dryer beforehand will make the after-shower experience nice, pleasant, and toasty.

Dressing Tips:

- Dress the worst first and undress the worst last, straighten the fabric as you go, loosen before you dress or undress. The "worst" refers to the parts of the body that aren't as flexible as the others.

Getting Through the Day Tips:

- A baby monitor works great for people who may need it. This way you can help them when they need it most and you don't wake them at the most inconvenient times.
- I always suggest bringing a second pair of shoes with more slip resistance and something as simple as a walker with a seat or wheelchair. You can keep it in the trunk of the car if you don't need it right away. Especially helpful if your Loved One can't stand for long periods of time.

Oral Care Tips:

- Always offer water every chance you can, though, some people are restricted water and moistening the mouth will help with their feeling of thirst.

- If you run out of dent-tips, use a wet paper towel around your finger or a toothbrush. It'll work just the same. Warning: Don't go into the teeth if you use your finger. You won't come back with it. Our bites are harder than you know with or without teeth.

When It's Over Tips:

- If your Loved One has a DNR and has stopped breathing, it is ok to take your time before calling hospice if you or your family requests extra time with your Loved One's body. But I suggest doing it in a timely fashion, considering nature will take its course and we all know what happens after.

Want to go Pro?

I am very proud that you are willing to put yourself out there to help others in time of need. I love you for that. The reward is great and you get paid to do what you love. The longer you do and the better you are, the better the reward and the greater the pay. However:

WARNING!

If caregiving is something you would like to do professionally, understand this is not just a "pays the bills" type of job. If you think you're going to "babysit" by sitting around and doing nothing, fire yourself now. Think twice before you jeopardize another and accept accountability for what you put your name on.

Whenever you think about how much stability you'll have, every day can be a rocking boat in the sea. You will be problem-solving for others all day, picking people up and having full responsibility in your hands. You can hurt people and God forbid the worse. Your fault. These are other people's lives we're talking about here. It is also not for the faint of the stomach. If you are easily grossed out and don't need a lot of activity, this may not be the job for you, but who knows. It may awaken your passion for being a better person and there for others.

Look into local caregiving courses and professional certificate classes that will help you receive the necessary training and credentials needed.

Have no fear; worry ends when your faith begins. Put it in the almighty high and yourself. You're his Sidekick for your life.

In Closing

Soiled Linens and Proud of it!

If you think this is a cruddy way to live life, then you have not acknowledged the love and gratitude that will be given to you when you do for others. See for yourself. Be proud of You and Yours.

You have someone who needs your help and in order to do that for them you need to follow your "Promise." Stick to it!

Well, this is the end. Despite a little hair loss and temporary writer's block, I really enjoyed writing this form of support for you.

Now you understand how to do it. Even better, you can see it from a professional's point of view in my own personal unwritten book of experience.

Well now it is written.

A Special Thank You

God, it is true! Through Christ and with a little patience on my part, YOU allow ALL things to become possible, I love you and thank you. Tell Momma Jackie and Mommy Ayin (My very FIRST reader) I said, "hi" and "I love them. I'm here with "Poopsie"

Daddy: I love you to the moon and back. Call you Sunday. My parents and grandparents showed me life philosophically and ethically, giving me a chance to see the world with open eyes and believe in myself. Family, I have too many of you to name. However, I love you all and thank you for being in my life. You have made me who I am today. But for my siblings. Josh and Joyce - Thank you for showing me what courage is. If you can take a leap of faith in your endeavors, so can I. I love you. Wesley, thank you for lighting a flame under my ass and making me give myself a deadline. Love you BUB! Thank you for giving me a new sister-in-law, Rachael and her daughter Annie. Krystal and Lore, if you didn't listen to me growing up in my most crazy times, I might have been in the asylum. Pab, thank you. It's a hard job and you're a perfect soul. Cindy (Cousin), you rock for being an important reader of mine. Thank you for the insight. My Aunts, Uncles and Cousins, I love you, Melonie, my best cousin. Aunt Tami thank you for being the God Mother I needed. Becca Bird, for reading it, I know it was a lot. Nieces and Nephews- I love you Booboo, Doo-doo, pooper, mac, Lil Katie, Lo-lo, Jake and Jonna. I love you guys.

Friends

Pat-Pat, fifteen years has been too long. I hope I made you proud. Thank you for starting this journey with me and I'm glad it was you; I love you. Nancy – Thank you. You are a wonderful artist with beautiful creativity and the world is brighter for it. Kristine, Judy – Thank you for your encouragement in this book and for telling me to put myself out there. Knuwane and Ellie- Love you, Lata Gals. Crystal and Isis, I love you and wish you the world. Amanda, I love you very much and I hope to hear from you. I hope someday we can have the chance to be friends again and I can be the friend you deserve. I'm sorry I wasn't the best friend to anyone, but you all have changed my life. I sincerely apologize to anyone I may have crossed paths with and offended. It was never my intention to cause anyone the slightest discomfort.

Laura Lee and Sue. I love you guys. Thank you for being there. Hi Lorraine, Love you, Boogoo, NIDA DANG! Hi Ivory, Ebony loves you— Anne "Nakupenda," Jesse "Mahal Kita," and all the rest of my posse. Yolanda Stewert, I wouldn't have gone down this road. God truly has an Angel in heaven.

I want to thank all my family and friends that I have made and who passed on; I love each and every one of you.

Light, you are the light that everyone should have had a chance to know. Rose- You and Jackie, the unit is in completion. I hope I live many years to come, but when my time arrives, I hope you come to welcome me with open arms.

My soulmate forever and a thousand times over, I don't see a full life of mine going by without you. You are the elephant I hold onto so dear and sacred enough to know you're my missing puzzle piece to unlock more love. You Complete me, my love, life, family, best friend, partner, ride or die. I love you always and for all eternity.

And a Very special thank you above ALL is to YOU! (God excluded) Thank you for doing your part as a human and caring for another who needs help. I love you for that. There is no better way to rid the world of separatism and hatred. You are doing the work God wants us to do. Be good or good at it, my friend.

About The Author

My name is K Rose Copeland and I am a Certified Nursing Assistant working for a Hospice. I live in Las Vegas, Nevada, with my spouse of fourteen years and two of the world's cutest cats.

I'm a jack of all trades, hopefully, a master of something.

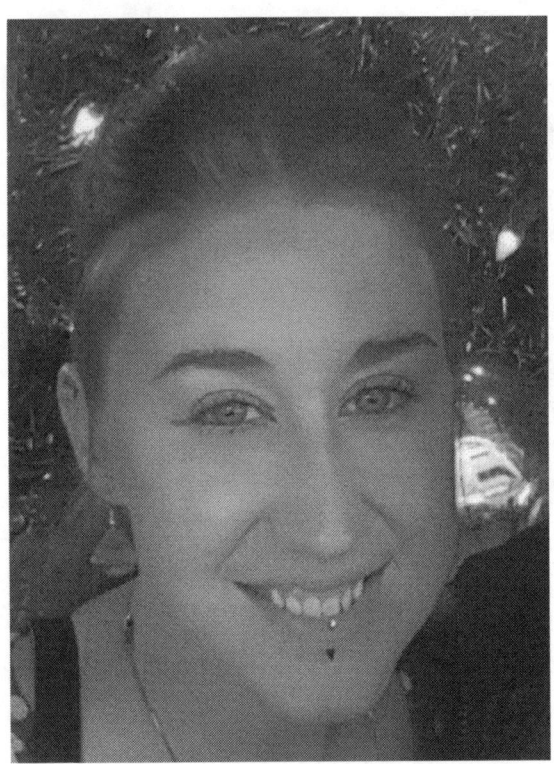

Disclaimer of Liability

The material and information contained in this book are for general informational purposes only. You should not only rely on the material contained in this book. Please seek medical advice before making any big decisions.

Nothing I said should be taken up the wazoo.

Made in the USA
Columbia, SC
15 October 2024

44377766R00137